TABLE OF CONTENTS

INTRODUCTION

This handbook serves a crucial role for anyone stepping into the realm of healthcare, providing a clear understanding of pathophysiology and the study of how disease processes affect the body. Why is this important? It's simple: every symptom and medical condition stems from an underlying biological cause. By mastering the concepts within these pages, you can trace symptoms back to their roots, understand the progression of diseases, and foresee potential complications. This knowledge sharpens your clinical acumen and enhances your ability to communicate with patients and other healthcare professionals about the why and how of medical conditions.

Pathophysiology forms the bridge between basic sciences and clinical practice. It's the core knowledge that informs all medical and therapeutic decisions. For a healthcare provider, understanding pathophysiology is akin to a detective understanding motives and methods in solving a crime. Without this insight, treatment can be a shot in the dark. With it, therapies become targeted, precise, and, most importantly, effective.

For instance, consider hypertension—a condition with various potential triggers, including genetic factors, lifestyle choices, and environmental influences. A firm grasp of pathophysiology allows a clinician to identify whether hypertension in a patient could be due to excess salt intake, stress, a genetic predisposition, or another cause. This understanding is crucial in choosing the right treatment strategy.

This handbook is designed not just to inform but also to be a practical guide in the clinic. It includes detailed descriptions of disease mechanisms, critical for medical students, and streamlined summaries useful for quick reference by practicing clinicians. The layout is intuitive, guiding you through each system of the body without the need to navigate through dense medical jargon.

With every chapter, you'll find that complex concepts are broken down into understandable segments. Each section builds upon the last, ensuring a cohesive learning experience. Whether reading straight through or dipping in to brush up on a specific area, you will find clear, practical, and relevant content to support your clinical decisions.

By the end of this handbook, your journey through the intricate landscape of human physiology and pathology will equip you with a comprehensive and nuanced toolkit, enhancing your capability to deliver high-quality care and improve patient outcomes.

This handbook is crafted to be an indispensable ally as a comprehensive guide and a quick reference during clinical rounds. Its design combines utility with simplicity, ensuring that whether you're a student or a seasoned clinician, the information you need is readily accessible and presented in an engaging and easy-to-navigate format.

As you explore the pages, you'll notice strategic highlights like quick reference symbols and critical terms. These aren't just markers; they're beacons, guiding you through the dense forest of medical jargon and complex concepts. A lightning bolt symbol, for example, signifies urgent actions and crucial points that demand your attention and are pivotal in clinical settings. A magnifying glass might encourage you to explore a topic further, enhancing your understanding.

The structure of the chapters is where this handbook truly excels. Each begins with a brief overview, setting the stage for what's to come. This isn't just an introduction; it's a roadmap outlining the journey through the intricacies of diseases and their underpinnings. As you move forward, you'll find a logical progression from the basics of each condition to the detailed aspects of clinical manifestations and management strategies. It's like following a narrative thread that educates and engages.

Step into this handbook not just to learn but to immerse yourself in pathophysiology in a format designed to cater to your learning needs. With each page turned, you're not just reading— you're becoming a more skilled and informed healthcare provider

CHAPTER 1:
CARDIOVASCULAR SYSTEM

Understanding the cardiovascular system and its pathophysiology is essential for anyone in the medical field. This section provides a clear view of how the heart and blood vessel functions can be disrupted by disease. Conditions such as atherosclerosis and hypertension are explored to explain how they lead to serious health issues like heart attacks or strokes. The content is structured to describe these diseases, focusing on their development, the underlying mechanisms that drive them, and the typical signs and symptoms observed in patients. This knowledge is crucial for effective diagnosis and management, helping healthcare professionals make informed decisions that can significantly impact patient outcomes.

Anatomy and Physiology of the Heart

The circulatory system's engine room is the heart, an essential organ. It circulates blood throughout the body, taking away waste materials and carbon dioxide while providing tissues with nutrition and oxygen. The heart is made up of two upper atria and two bottom ventricles, or chambers, structurally. The myocardium, its specialized muscle, contracts continuously and rhythmically throughout life.

Key Pathophysiological Processes

Atherosclerosis and hypertension are two pathophysiological processes that demonstrate how cardiovascular health might be jeopardized. Fatty deposits accumulate within the arteries as a result of atherosclerosis. The arteries may become narrowed and hardened by these plaques, which would decrease blood flow and raise the risk of heart attacks and strokes. High blood pressure, often known as hypertension, puts additional strain on the heart by making it work harder to pump blood. This increasing effort over time may cause the heart muscle to thicken and ultimately result in heart failure.

The way both disorders impact the arteries and shared risk factors like smoking, inactivity, and poor nutrition are what connect them. Comprehending these mechanisms is essential for prevention and treatment, emphasizing alterations in lifestyle and prescription drugs to regulate blood pressure and cholesterol levels. With this knowledge, patients may take proactive steps to preserve heart health and healthcare professionals can deliver tailored therapies.

Critical Conditions and Management:

Maintaining cardiovascular health requires managing severe illnesses such as hypertension and myocardial infarction through a mix of lifestyle modifications and medication. Hypertension, characterized by persistently high blood pressure, necessitates adjustments such as reduced salt intake, regular physical activity, and stress management. Medications may include beta- blockers or ACE inhibitors to control blood pressure effectively.

A heart attack, sometimes referred to as a myocardial infarction, need prompt medical attention. Treatment focuses on restoring blood flow to the heart, often through medications like aspirin and more advanced procedures such as angioplasty. Following a heart attack, long- term management includes medications to prevent clots, reduce heart workload, and stabilize heart rhythms.

The key to treating these problems is quitting smoking, maintaining a heart-healthy diet, and getting regular exercise. Treatment effectiveness and the avoidance of problems are greatly aided by early diagnosis and timely medical attention. This strategy lowers the likelihood of serious consequences like heart failure or stroke while simultaneously improving quality of life.

Hypertension:

High blood pressure, often known as hypertension, is a frequent illness where the blood's force on the artery walls is so great that it may eventually lead to health issues including heart disease. In order to delay the development of more serious consequences such as renal damage, heart attack, and stroke, hypertension must

8

be properly managed.

A multifaceted approach is often required to manage hypertension effectively. Lifestyle changes are foundational; among them are cutting back on cholesterol, saturated fats, and salt in the diet. Including healthy grains, fruits, and veggies in your everyday meals can have a big impact. It is advised to engage in regular physical activity, such as 30 minutes of moderate exercise, most days of the week in order to naturally reduce blood pressure. Additionally, reducing alcohol consumption and quitting smoking are crucial steps, as both can elevate blood pressure.

For many individuals, lifestyle adjustments need to be supplemented with medication. Commonly prescribed medications include:

- *Diuretics aid in the body's salt elimination by the kidneys.*
- *With ACE inhibitors, blood vessels are relaxed.*
- *Beta-blockers to lower blood flow and heart rate.*
- *To guarantee ideal blood pressure management and make any therapy adjustments, regular monitoring by a healthcare professional is crucial*

Etiology

Based on its origin, hypertension may be divided into two types: main and secondary. Primary hypertension, also known as essential hypertension, is the most common type and does not have a clear cause. But it usually takes years to manifest and is associated with poor nutrition, age, genetics, and inactivity. On the other hand, secondary hypertension can develop unexpectedly and has a known etiology. It is linked to underlying medical issues such renal illness, endocrine abnormalities, congenital cardiac defects, or drug usage. Understanding whether hypertension is primary or secondary is crucial for determining the most effective treatment strategy. In situations of secondary hypertension, this entails treating any underlying diseases that may be causing high blood pressure in addition to controlling blood pressure with medication and lifestyle changes.

Pathophysiological Mechanisms

The complicated pathophysiological mechanisms behind hypertension include several bodily systems, most notably the Sympathetic Nervous System (SNS) and the Renin-Angiotensin-Aldosterone System (RAAS).

In order to maintain fluid balance and control blood pressure, the RAAS is essential. When the blood pressure drops or the kidneys sense a decrease in blood flow, the enzyme renin is produced. The liver-produced protein angiotensinogen is then transformed by renin into angiotensin I, which is ultimately transformed into angiotensin II by the lungs' angiotensin- converting enzyme (ACE). Strong vasoconstrictor angiotensin II causes blood vessels to narrow and blood pressure to rise. Additionally, it causes the adrenal glands to secrete more aldosterone, which causes the kidneys to retain water and salt and raises blood pressure even more.

Overactivity of the SNS also contributes to hypertension. This system can increase heart rate and contractility, narrow blood vessels, and stimulate renin release through adrenergic receptors. Chronic stress, lifestyle factors, and genetic predispositions can lead to sustained SNS activation, which elevates blood pressure persistently.

Together, these mechanisms demonstrate how various factors and bodily systems interplay to regulate blood pressure, which, when dysregulated, can lead to hypertension.

Clinical Signs

Elevated blood pressure is the primary clinical sign of hypertension, which often prompts investigation. This is typically identified during routine checks using a sphygmomanometer, which measures the pressure in the arteries at various heart cycle phases. Readings consistently above 130/80 mmHg are generally considered hypertensive and may necessitate further evaluation and management.

In addition to raising blood pressure, hypertension can harm organs. This term refers to damage to major organs fed by the circulatory system, primarily due to prolonged elevated blood pressure. This covers the kidneys, brain, eyes, and heart. It can cause hypertensive heart disease, which can lead to heart failure in the end as well as left ventricular hypertrophy and coronary artery disease. The kidneys may suffer from nephrosclerosis, decreasing their ability to filter waste and balance fluids, electrolytes, and acids. In the brain, the excessive pressure can lead to strokes and cognitive impairment. Hypertensive retinopathy, where high blood pressure damages the vessels of the retina, affecting vision, is another critical concern.

These signs underscore the importance of managing blood pressure within a healthy range to prevent serious complications and improve overall health outcomes.

Diagnostic Criteria: JNC 8 Guidelines, BP Measurement Techniques

The diagnosis of hypertension largely follows the JNC 8 guidelines, which provide specific criteria based on blood pressure measurements. Per these criteria, a person is diagnosed with hypertension if their blood pressure regularly registers at 140/90 mmHg or higher for the general population, or 130/80 mmHg or above for individuals who have chronic renal disease or diabetes.

Techniques for measuring blood pressure are essential for precise diagnosis. Using a sphygmomanometer that has been correctly calibrated and certified is crucial. With their feet on the floor and their arms at heart level, the patient should sit quietly on a chair for at least five minutes. It is advised to take several readings at least twice in order to confirm the diagnosis of hypertension. An automated instrument, mercury, or aneroid manometer can be used to manually take these measurements.

Reliability of measurements is ensured by proper procedure, which is essential for accurately diagnosing and treating hypertension. Frequent monitoring lowers the risk of problems connected to hypertension by assisting in the adjustment of medications to reach and maintain appropriate blood pressure levels.

Management

Effective hypertension management combines lifestyle changes with first-line antihypertensive drugs when necessary. Lifestyle changes are the foundation of hypertension management and can significantly reduce blood pressure. Eating well is very beneficial, especially when following the Dietary Approaches to Stop Hypertension (DASH) diet. This diet limits added sugars, cholesterol, and saturated fats while emphasizing fruits, vegetables, whole grains, lean meats, and low-fat dairy. It is crucial to limit sodium consumption to less than 2,300 mg (or 1,500 mg for individuals at higher risk) per day, which may be accomplished by avoiding processed foods and using less salt while cooking.

Frequent exercise, like 150 minutes a week of moderate exercise (such brisk walking and cycling), helps control blood pressure and help people maintain a healthy weight. Reducing alcohol intake, giving up smoking, and engaging in stress-relieving activities like yoga, meditation, or deep breathing all help to maintain blood pressure management.

When lifestyle changes alone are insufficient, first-line antihypertensive medications are introduced. ACE inhibitors, such as lisinopril, relax blood arteries and are especially useful for diabetic patients. Calcium channel blockers, such as amlodipine, are frequently used by older persons to lower blood pressure by relaxing arteries. By encouraging the excretion of water and salt, thiazide diuretics (such as hydrochlorothiazide) lower blood volume and consequently blood pressure. When ACE inhibitors are intolerable, ARBs (like losartan) act as stand-ins by inhibiting angiotensin II at the receptor level.

To get the best possible control, a mix of drugs that target different systems involved in blood pressure management is frequently required. Regular follow-up with healthcare providers ensures ongoing monitoring and adjustments in treatment and reinforces the importance of lifestyle changes. This all-encompassing strategy lowers the risk of consequences including heart attack, stroke, and renal disease by successfully managing blood pressure.

Myocardial Infarction (MI):

A myocardial infarction (MI), sometimes referred to as a heart attack, happens when blood supply is cut off to a portion of the heart for an extended period of time, causing damage or even death to a portion of the heart muscle. The most common cause of this is a plaque (a mixture of fat, cholesterol, and other materials) blockage in one or more coronary arteries. These plaques have the potential to burst, causing a blood clot to restrict blood flow.

A heart attack's common symptoms include pain or discomfort in the chest that might radiate to the arm, jaw, mouth, or back. Heartburn, nausea, indigestion, and stomach discomfort are possible additional symptoms. Breathlessness, chills, exhaustion, and abrupt lightheadedness are typical symptoms.

Immediate treatment for MI is critical to minimize heart damage. Treatments include medication such as aspirin and thrombolytics, which dissolve clots and restore blood flow. In some cases, procedures like angioplasty, where the blocked artery is mechanically widened, or coronary artery bypass surgery, where the blood is rerouted around a blocked artery, are required.

Preventing MI involves:

- *Modifying one's lifestyle to reduce risk factors, for as by eating a balanced diet.*
- *Engaging in regular exercise.*
- *Staying away from tobacco smoke.*
- *Keeping a healthy weight in mind.*

Prescription drugs may also be used to treat illnesses like high blood pressure or hypercholesterolemia, which raise the risk of a heart attack.

Pathophysiology

The most frequent cause of myocardial infarction (MI), sometimes referred to as a heart attack, is the coronary arteries' atherosclerotic plaque rupturing. This rupture exposes the contents of the plaque to blood, initiating the clotting process. Platelets and clotting factors accumulate rapidly at the site, forming a thrombus obstructing blood flow. This blockage deprives heart muscle cells of oxygen, causing tissue damage or death, a condition known as ischemia. The severity of the heart attack depends on the clot's size and how long the artery remains blocked. In order to minimize cardiac damage and break the clot and restore blood flow, prompt medical intervention is essential.

Clinical Presentation

When a myocardial infarction (MI), sometimes referred to as a heart attack, manifests clinically, it usually causes chest pain or discomfort that is felt as fullness, pressure, or squeezing in the middle of the chest. The jaw, neck, back, shoulders, and arms may all feel the same pain. Dyspnea, or shortness of breath, is a common accompanying symptom that can happen either before or after the chest discomfort. Other symptoms include a chilly sweat, nausea, and dizziness. Early intervention can greatly improve the prognosis for heart attack victims, but prompt diagnosis of these signs is essential.

Diagnostic Workup

The diagnostic workup for a myocardial infarction (MI) typically involves an electrocardiogram (ECG) and measurement of cardiac biomarkers. An ECG can detect changes in the heart's electrical activity, indicating areas of muscle damage. T-wave inversions, ST-elevation, or the creation of a new left bundle branch block are examples of fundamental modifications. Cardiac biomarkers, proteins released into the blood from damaged heart cells, are also crucial for diagnosis. The most commonly measured biomarkers are troponins, which are highly specific to heart injury. Elevated levels can confirm a heart attack, even when there are no apparent symptoms or ECG changes.

Acute Management

Acute myocardial infarction (MI) management often follows the MONA protocol: Aspirin, nitroglycerin, oxygen, and morphine. In order to treat excruciating chest pain and lessen cardiac strain, morphine is injected. If the patient's blood oxygen level is low, oxygen is administered to enhance oxygen delivery to the heart tissue. By widening blood arteries, nitroglycerin lessens the burden on the heart and increases blood flow. Aspirin is an essential component of the treatment because it thins the blood and stops further blood clotting, which lowers the chance of the coronary artery blockage getting worse.

Long-Term Management

Improving heart function and lowering the risk of further cardiac events are the main goals of long-term therapy of myocardial infarction (MI). Beta-blockers are commonly prescribed as they reduce the heart's workload and prevent abnormal heart rhythms, which can lower the risk of further attacks. By helping to relax blood arteries, ACE inhibitors lower the risk of heart failure and facilitate the heart's ability to pump blood. By reducing cholesterol, statins can help stop new plaque from accumulating in the arteries. Together, these medications form a critical part of ongoing care for patients recovering from a heart attack.

Heart Failure

When the heart cannot adequately pump blood to satisfy the body's demands, heart failure results. It may be brought on by illnesses including hypertension, coronary artery disease, or cardiac muscle weakening following a prior heart attack. Systolic (lower pumping capacity) and diastolic (poor filling capacity) heart failures are different from one another. Breathlessness, exhaustion, leg swelling, and fluid retention are some of the symptoms. To enhance heart function and quality of life, management entails modifying lifestyle habits and using drugs such as beta-blockers to lessen heart strain, ACE inhibitors to relax blood vessels, and diuretics to prevent fluid accumulation.

Types: Systolic vs. Diastolic Dysfunction

The two main categories of heart failure are diastolic and systolic dysfunction. Heart failure with reduced ejection fraction (HFrEF), commonly referred to as systolic dysfunction, is the result of the left ventricle's inability to contract efficiently. Because of this dysfunction, the heart is unable to pump enough blood to satisfy the body's requirements. The amount of blood the left ventricle pumps out with each contraction is measured by the ejection fraction, which is lowered in HFrEF. This reduction results in insufficient circulation, which causes symptoms such as exhaustion, dyspnea, and fluid build-up in the lungs and legs.

Heart failure with preserved ejection fraction, also known as diastolic dysfunction (HFpEF), occurs when the heart stiffens and is unable to relax sufficiently in between beats. Although the heart can still contract normally, its stiffness prevents it from filling with enough blood during the resting phase. Consequently, the amount of blood pumped out in each heartbeat may be sufficient, but the overall volume is reduced due to the heart's inability to fill correctly. HFpEF often leads to symptoms like shortness of breath, especially during exertion, and fluid retention in the lungs and extremities.

The symptoms of both forms of heart failure might be similar, including exhaustion, swelling in the legs, and trouble breathing. But different underlying systems affect how they are managed. In HFrEF, treatment focuses on medications that improve the heart's pumping ability, like ACE inhibitors, beta-blockers, and diuretics. In HFpEF, managing blood pressure, addressing comorbidities like diabetes, and using diuretics to control fluid retention are primary strategies. While both conditions share some treatment approaches, understanding whether the dysfunction is systolic or diastolic helps tailor therapy to the patient's specific heart failure type, aiming for the best possible outcomes.

Pathophysiological Mechanisms: Ventricular Remodeling, Fluid Overload

In heart failure, two fundamental pathophysiological mechanisms are ventricular remodeling and fluid overload. When the heart muscle undergoes persistent stress or damage—such as during a heart attack—it can alter in size, shape, and function. This condition is known as ventricular remodeling. The heart's pumping efficiency may be decreased by enlargement and thickening of the walls. Fluid overload results from the heart's inability to maintain proper blood circulation, causing fluid to go back into the lungs, abdomen, and legs. This fluid retention contributes to symptoms like swelling, shortness of breath, and weight gain, worsening the strain on the weakened heart.

Key Signs: Dyspnea, Edema, JVD (Jugular Venous Distention)

Dyspnea, edema, and jugular venous distention are important indicators of heart failure (JVD). Breathing becomes difficult for the patient with dyspnea, or shortness of breath, especially while they are lying down or engaging in physical activity. This condition is frequently caused by fluid accumulation in the lungs. Edema is the swelling that develops in the legs, ankles, and feet as a result of fluid buildup in the tissues brought on by the heart's ineffective blood pumping mechanism.

A noticeable enlargement of the veins in the neck, known as jugular venous distention (JVD), denotes elevated pressure in the venous system. Blood backs up in the veins as a result of the heart's inability to pump blood through the circulatory system

20

properly. These symptoms are essential for identifying heart failure and determining how serious it is. This information informs management and therapy plans aimed at enhancing the patient's quality of life.

Diagnostics: Echocardiography, BNP Levels

Diagnosing heart failure involves several vital tests, with echocardiography and measurement of BNP (B-type Natriuretic Peptide) levels being among the most important. A non-invasive imaging procedure called echocardiography employs ultrasonic pulses to produce finely detailed images of the heart. It allows healthcare providers to assess the heart's structure and function, including the heart chambers' size and shape, the heart muscle's thickness, and how well the heart pumps blood. Finding out if the heart failure is diastolic (maintained ejection fraction) or systolic (lower ejection fraction) can be better achieved using this test. It also helps identify other potential causes of symptoms, such as valve problems or abnormal blood flow.

The hormone known as BNP, or B-type Natriuretic Peptide, is produced by the heart in reaction to elevated intra-cardiac pressure. BNP levels increase in heart failure because the heart has to work harder to pump blood, which causes the heart muscle to stretch. Measuring BNP levels through a blood test can help confirm a diagnosis of heart failure, especially when symptoms like shortness of breath and swelling are present. Elevated BNP levels strongly indicate heart failure and can also provide insight into the severity of the condition.

Together, echocardiography and BNP testing provide a comprehensive evaluation of heart function. Echocardiography visually assesses the heart's mechanics, while BNP levels offer biochemical evidence of the heart's stress and workload. These tests are crucial for verifying heart failure, assessing its severity, and recommending the best course of action. They also assist in keeping an eye on how well treatments are working and modifying management tactics as needed to enhance patient results.

Management: Diuretics, ACE Inhibitors, Lifestyle Modifications

In order to reduce symptoms, halt the course of the condition, and enhance overall quality of life, heart failure must be managed with a mix of medicines and lifestyle modifications. Diuretics, sometimes referred to as "water pills," are an essential component of care. They lessen swelling (edema) and lessen the strain on the heart by assisting the kidneys in eliminating extra fluid and salt from the body. Diuretics also help alleviate shortness of breath, a common symptom in heart failure patients, by preventing fluid buildup in the lungs.

ACE inhibitors are another critical component of heart failure management. These drugs function by decreasing blood pressure, widening blood arteries, and lightening the heart's pumping effort. They aid in halting further ventricular remodeling, which over time may exacerbate heart failure. ACE inhibitors can significantly reduce symptoms and enhance patient outcomes by improving blood flow and decreasing strain on the heart.

Changes in lifestyle are equally significant. Patients are advised to eat a low-sodium diet since too much salt might exacerbate symptoms and cause fluid retention. It is advised to engage in regular, moderate exercise to strengthen the heart and enhance circulation. Reducing alcohol consumption and giving up smoking can also improve heart health. Monitoring weight daily helps identify rapid fluid accumulation, allowing for early intervention. Medications and lifestyle changes form a practical approach to managing heart failure, focusing on symptom relief and preventing further complications.

Quick Clinical Assessment Checklist

A quick clinical assessment for heart failure is crucial to identify key symptoms and signs for timely management. Vital indicators such as blood pressure, heart rate, breathing rate, and oxygen saturation can be measured to determine the general state of the cardiovascular system. Worsening cardiac function may be indicated by low blood pressure or an elevated heart rate. It's crucial to enquire about symptoms from patients, such as breathing difficulties after exercise or while lying down, sudden weight gain, abdominal or leg edema, and ongoing exhaustion.

During the physical examination, observe for swelling in the legs and ankles, and check the neck for signs of jugular venous distention. Listen to the lungs for crackles, which could indicate fluid buildup. Additionally, monitoring changes in the patient's weight is essential, as sudden increases may suggest fluid retention. This straightforward assessment helps recognize heart failure symptoms early and guides appropriate interventions.

Vital Signs: BP, Pulse

Keeping an eye on vital indicators like blood pressure (BP) and pulse is essential for determining how well a patient with heart failure is doing. Blood pressure readings provide insight into how well the heart is pumping and if there is excessive strain on the cardiovascular system. In heart failure, blood pressure may vary, often elevated in earlier stages due to compensatory mechanisms or becoming low as the condition worsens, indicating a weakened heart.

Pulse rate and rhythm are equally important. A rapid or irregular pulse can suggest that the heart works harder to maintain circulation, which might indicate worsening heart function. Regular monitoring of these vital signs aids in assessing the efficacy of therapy and enables required modifications to drug or management regimens. Frequent monitoring of blood pressure and pulse gives a comprehensive picture of the patient's cardiovascular health and helps with treatment decision-making for heart failure.

Red Flags for Immediate Action

Specific symptoms and signs of heart failure require immediate attention to prevent serious complications. Rapid weight gain, usually more than two to three pounds daily or five pounds weekly, can indicate sudden fluid retention. Severe shortness of breath, mainly if it occurs at rest or worsens significantly, may point to acute pulmonary edema, which demands prompt intervention.

Chest pain or tightness, especially if it radiates to the arms or jaw, could signal a heart attack. Dizziness, fainting, or confusion might indicate reduced blood flow to the brain, suggesting worsening heart failure. These red flags require urgent medical evaluation and action to stabilize the patient and adjust treatment as necessary.

CHAPTER 2: RESPIRATORY SYSTEM

The respiratory system is in charge of taking carbon dioxide out of the body, which is a waste product of metabolism, and giving the organism oxygen. Pathophysiology in this system arises when diseases or conditions disrupt these processes, affecting the lungs, airways, or respiratory muscles. This disruption can lead to reduced oxygen intake and impaired gas exchange, resulting in shortness of breath, coughing, wheezing, and decreased exercise tolerance.

Restriction lung diseases, pneumonia, asthma, and chronic obstructive pulmonary disease (COPD) are common respiratory pathologies. These conditions involve various mechanisms, such as inflammation, airway obstruction, alveolar damage, and loss of lung elasticity. Understanding the pathophysiological changes in the respiratory system is essential for diagnosing, managing, and improving the outcomes of patients with respiratory disorders.

Basic Anatomy and Physiology of the Lungs

The ribcage surrounds the two spongy organs that make up the lungs in the chest. They are essential to breathing because they make it easier for the blood to exchange carbon dioxide and oxygen with the surrounding air. Through the mouth or nose, air enters the body and passes through the trachea, bronchi, and tiny bronchioles inside each lung. Alveoli are microscopic air sacs where these bronchioles terminate.

Gas exchange takes place in the alveoli, which are surrounded by a network of capillaries. While carbon dioxide travels from the blood into the alveoli to be expelled, oxygen travels through the thin walls of the alveoli and into the blood. During breathing, the diaphragm and intercostal muscles help to expand and contract the lungs, maintaining a constant flow of air. The effective operation of this system is essential for keeping the body's oxygen levels stable and eliminating carbon dioxide.

Key Pathophysiological Processes

Key pathophysiological processes in the respiratory system include obstruction, restriction, and inflammation. Conditions such as asthma and chronic obstructive pulmonary disease (COPD) are characterized by obstructive processes. These happen when bronchoconstriction, excessive mucus production, or structural abnormalities in the airway walls cause the airways to narrow or become clogged.

This leads to difficulty exhaling air, resulting in symptoms like wheezing, coughing, and shortness of breath.

Restrictive processes involve a reduction in lung expansion, often due to stiffness in lung tissue or the chest wall. Conditions like pulmonary fibrosis cause scarring of lung tissue, making the lungs less elastic and more difficult to inflate. Restrictive issues can also result from neuromuscular disorders or structural abnormalities, limiting lung volumes and reducing oxygen intake.

Inflammation plays a central role in many respiratory diseases. It leads to swelling of the airways, increased mucus production, and damage to lung tissue. In asthma, for example, inflammation results in hyperresponsiveness of the airways, triggering episodes of bronchoconstriction. Pneumonia and other infections inflame the lung tissue, impairing gas exchange and producing symptoms including fever, coughing, and dyspnea. It is essential to understand these mechanisms in order to properly diagnose and treat respiratory disorders.

Critical Conditions and Management:

Asthma, pneumonia, and chronic obstructive pulmonary disease (COPD) are examples of critical respiratory disorders. Improving patient outcomes and quality of life requires effective care of these disorders.

The inflammatory and hyperresponsive airways that result from asthma cause bronchoconstriction, mucus accumulation, and symptoms including coughing, wheezing, and shortness of breath. Controlling inflammation and avoiding acute episodes are the main goals of treatment. Short-acting beta-agonists (SABA), one type of quick-relief drug, relax the muscles in the airways to produce relief right away. Inhaled corticosteroids, for example, are long-term control drugs that lower inflammation and stop symptoms.

COPD is a progressive lung disease primarily caused by smoking. It involves chronic airway obstruction and alveolar damage. Management aims to alleviate symptoms, slow disease progression, and prevent exacerbations. Airway opening is facilitated by bronchodilators, such as beta-agonists and anticholinergics. Programs for pulmonary rehabilitation enhance lung function and exercise tolerance, while inhaled corticosteroids lessen inflammation.

Respiratory infections, like pneumonia, result in inflammation and fluid accumulation in the lungs. Management includes antibiotics for bacterial infections, antivirals if a virus is a cause, and supportive care like oxygen therapy and fluids. Timely identification and treatment are crucial to preventing complications and ensuring effective recovery.

Asthma:

The chronic illness known as asthma is characterized by inflammation and hyperresponsiveness of the airways, which can result in bouts of bronchoconstriction. Wheezing, shortness of breath, chest tightness, and coughing are common symptoms that are frequently brought on by allergies, physical activity, cold air, or stress.

Breathing becomes challenging due to the swelling and overproduction of mucus in the airways. The main goals of management are to stop attacks and reduce inflammation. Short-acting beta-agonists (SABA) are used as quick-relief drugs to relieve symptoms immediately; inhaled corticosteroids are utilized for long-term management to lower airway inflammation. Another important strategy for reducing the frequency and intensity of asthma flare-ups is to recognize and stay away from triggers.

Pathophysiology: Bronchoconstriction, Inflammation

Asthma's pathophysiology involves two main processes: bronchoconstriction and inflammation. During an asthma episode, exposure to triggers like allergens, cold air, exercise, or irritants causes the airways to react abnormally. Bronchoconstriction, a narrowing of the airways and difficulty breathing, is caused by the smooth muscles surrounding the bronchi constricting or tightening. Breathlessness, tightness in the chest, and wheezing are the results of this procedure.

The underlying chronic mechanism in asthma is inflammation. Eosinophils, mast cells, and T lymphocytes are examples of inflammatory cells that penetrate the airway walls and release chemicals that result in swelling and mucus formation. The thickened airway walls further restrict airflow, contributing to the feeling of breathlessness. This ongoing inflammation makes the airways hyperresponsive, easily triggered by factors that would not affect healthy lungs. If persistent inflammation is not well controlled, it might eventually cause remodeling—structural alterations in the airways—which can deteriorate lung function.

Managing asthma requires a dual approach: controlling the inflammation with long-term medications like inhaled corticosteroids to reduce swelling and bronchodilators to relieve acute bronchoconstriction. This approach helps maintain open airways, reduce symptoms, and prevent future asthma attacks.

Clinical Features: Wheezing, Shortness of Breath, Cough

The symptoms of asthma are unique and include coughing, shortness of breath, and wheezing. A high-pitched whistling sound caused by restricted airways that is audible when breathing, especially when expelling, is called wheezing. This airway constriction symptom is frequently the most identifiable one associated with asthma.

As the airways get more irritated and constricted, it becomes more difficult for air to enter and exit the lungs, resulting in shortness of breath. This can cause chest tightness and make it difficult to breathe deeply, particularly while engaging in vigorous activity or being among triggers.

Coughing is another important symptom, especially in the early morning or late at night. It may be accompanied by thick, sticky mucous and is frequently persistent. The cough results from the body's effort to clear mucus from the inflamed airways. Recognizing these symptoms is essential for diagnosing and managing asthma effectively.

Diagnostic Tools: Peak Flow Meter, Spirometry

Diagnosing asthma involves using specific tools to measure lung function and airway responsiveness. Two essential diagnostic tools commonly used are the peak flow meter and spirometry.

A small, basic instrument called a peak flow meter calculates the fastest possible exhalation rate. It assesses how quickly air can be pushed out of the lungs, indicating airway constriction. Patients blow into the meter with as much force as possible, and the device records the peak expiratory flow rate (PEFR). Peak flow monitoring on a regular basis aids in the tracking of asthma management and the early detection of asthma attack symptoms by patients and healthcare professionals. A significant drop in peak flow readings may signal worsening inflammation or bronchoconstriction, allowing for timely intervention.

Spirometry, on the other hand, offers a more detailed assessment of lung function. Patients take a deep breath and exhale forcefully into the spirometer during the test. This apparatus measures vital signs like forced vital capacity (FVC) and forced expiratory volume in one second (FEV1). When diagnosing asthma, the FEV1/FVC ratio is essential since a lower ratio denotes airway restriction. Additionally useful in determining the severity of asthma and tracking the course of therapy response is spirometry. After administering a bronchodilator, an increase in FEV1

32

suggests reversible airway obstruction, a hallmark of asthma.

Peak flow measurement and spirometry provide valuable insights into airway function, guiding diagnosis and management. While the peak flow meter is helpful for daily self-monitoring, spirometry offers a more comprehensive evaluation, helping to confirm the diagnosis and tailor treatment plans. Regular use of these tools allows for early detection of changes in airway function, enabling effective asthma control and reducing the risk of acute attacks.

Acute Management: Short-acting Beta Agonists (SABA), Corticosteroids

Acute asthma management focuses on quickly relieving symptoms and preventing the condition from worsening. For asthma attacks, short-acting beta agonists (SABA) are the first line of therapy. These drugs, including albuterol, cause bronchodilation and better airflow by quickly relaxing the smooth muscles around the airways. Typically, patients use a nebulizer or a metered-dose inhaler to inhale these drugs to ease symptoms such as tightness in the chest, wheezing, and shortness of breath. SABAs have a minute half-life, which makes them crucial for treating acute symptoms.

Corticosteroids are another crucial component of acute management. When asthma symptoms are severe or do not respond adequately to SABA, oral or intravenous corticosteroids like prednisone are administered. These medications reduce inflammation in the airways, decreasing swelling and mucus production, which helps restore normal breathing. Unlike SABAs, corticosteroids take a few hours to show effects, but they are essential for controlling the underlying inflammation that drives the asthma attack and preventing a recurrence.

Together, using SABAs for immediate relief and corticosteroids for controlling inflammation forms an effective strategy for managing acute asthma episodes and minimizing the risk of complications.

Long-Term Management

Long-term asthma management is centered on controlling inflammation and preventing symptoms to maintain good respiratory function. For continued asthma management, inhaled corticosteroids (ICS) are the most effective drug.They directly reduce inflammation in the airways, decreasing swelling, mucus production, and sensitivity to triggers. Frequent usage of inhaled corticosteroids (ICS) like fluticasone or budesonide helps maintain open airways, reduces the frequency and intensity of asthma episodes, and enhances lung function overall. Unlike medications for immediate relief, ICS are taken daily, even when symptoms are absent, to maintain consistent control over the condition.

Leukotriene modifiers, such as montelukast, offer another approach for long-term asthma management. These medications block the action of leukotrienes, chemicals in the body that cause airway constriction, inflammation, and increased mucus production. By reducing the effects of leukotrienes, these drugs help prevent asthma symptoms and improvisation, especially in patients who experience symptoms triggered by allergies or exercise. Leukotriene modifiers are usually taken orally and can be used alongside inhaled corticosteroids for enhanced control.

Leukotriene modifiers and inhaled corticosteroids work synergistically to provide a customized strategy for maintaining asthma stability and lowering the incidence of acute exacerbations.

Chronic Obstructive Pulmonary Disease (COPD)

The progressive lung disease known as chronic obstructive pulmonary disease (COPD) is marked by a continuous restriction of airflow. It includes ailments like chronic bronchitis and emphysema, which are mostly brought on by prolonged exposure to irritants like cigarette smoke. The airways and alveoli are harmed in COPD, which results in a persistent cough, copious mucus production, and dyspnea. Breathing becomes more difficult when lungs lose their flexibility with age. The goal of management is to reduce the course of the illness and relieve symptoms by using bronchodilators, inhaled corticosteroids, pulmonary rehabilitation, and quitting smoking. The quality of life for COPD patients can be significantly improved with early diagnosis and diligent care.

Pathophysiology

The pathophysiology of COPD is primarily based on airflow restriction and alveolar damage. Chronic exposure to allergens, including tobacco smoke, causes the airways to become inflamed. Airflow obstruction results from this inflammation's thickening of the bronchial walls, increased mucus production, and constriction of the airways. The obstruction primarily affects exhalation, causing air to become trapped in the lungs and difficulty breathing.

Alveolar destruction occurs in emphysema, where the tiny air sacs responsible for gas exchange are damaged and lose their elasticity. This injury diminishes the surface area available for the exchange of oxygen and carbon dioxide, so compromising lung function and exacerbating symptoms such as persistent dyspnea and persistent coughing.

Clinical Features

COPD presents with several distinct clinical features, including chronic cough, sputum production, and dyspnea. The cough is usually persistent and often worse in the mornings. It may initially be intermittent but becomes more frequent as the disease progresses.

Sputum production is another hallmark of COPD. Due to chronic inflammation, the airways produce excess mucus, leading to frequent throat clearing and expectoration of sputum, which can be thick and vary in color.

Dyspnea, or shortness of breath, is a critical symptom that worsens over time. It often starts during physical activities, such as climbing stairs, but can eventually occur even at rest. This persistent breathlessness significantly impacts daily life and is primarily why patients seek medical attention.

Diagnostic Criteria

The diagnosis of COPD relies on specific criteria, primarily measured through spirometry. The forced expiratory volume in one second (FEV1) compared to the forced vital capacity (FVC) of the lungs is the important indication, or FEV1/FVC ratio. This ratio is less than 0.70 in COPD, which indicates ongoing airway restriction.

Based on the FEV1 measurement, the Global Initiative for Chronic Obstructive Lung Disease (GOLD) classifies the severity of COPD. The phases are modest (GOLD 1) to severe (GOLD 4), with more impairment indicated by lower FEV1 percentages. This categorization aids in directing patient care and treatment plans.

Management

Relieving symptoms, boosting lung function, and increasing quality of life are the main goals of COPD management. The mainstay of therapy is bronchodilators, which ease airflow and lessen dyspnea by relaxing the muscles around the airways. These drugs can be either long-acting, which offers more prolonged symptom management, or short-acting, which offers immediate relief.

Common bronchodilators include beta-agonists and anticholinergics, often delivered via inhalers or nebulizers. Pulmonary rehabilitation is another crucial aspect of management. It involves a structured program of exercise training, education, and breathing techniques designed to strengthen the respiratory muscles, improve physical endurance, and reduce symptoms. This approach helps patients manage their condition more effectively, enhancing their ability to perform daily activities and improving overall well-being.

Respiratory Infections (Pneumonia, Bronchitis)

For those who have COPD, respiratory infections like pneumonia and bronchitis are serious concerns since they can worsen the underlying disease and have serious consequences.

An illness known as pneumonia causes inflammation of one or both lungs' air sacs, which can then fill with pus or fluid. This results in symptoms including fever, chills, coughing up pus or mucus, and trouble breathing. Patients with COPD may be especially vulnerable to pneumonia, which raises the possibility of sudden respiratory failure.

The bronchial tube, which transports air to and from the lungs, becomes inflamed when someone has bronchitis. Coughing up mucous, wheezing, dyspnea, and a constriction in the chest are among the symptoms. While acute bacterial bronchitis can have serious negative effects on health, chronic bronchitis is frequently a hallmark of COPD.

Antibiotics are usually used to treat the bacterial origins of these illnesses, while bronchodilators and corticosteroids are used more often to reduce inflammation and facilitate breathing. It is also advised that individuals with COPD take preventative steps to lower their chance of contracting infections like pneumonia and influenza.

Common Pathogens: Bacterial vs. Viral Infections

Both bacterial and viral pathogens can cause respiratory infections, affecting the body differently.

Bacterial infections in the respiratory system often lead to bacterial pneumonia and acute bronchitis. Common bacterial pathogens include Streptococcus pneumonia, a leading cause of bacterial pneumonia, and Haemophilus influenza, which can cause both pneumonia and exacerbations of chronic bronchitis in COPD patients. Antibiotics effectively treat bacterial infections, targeting the specific pathogens responsible for the illness.

Viruses like the influenza virus, rhinoviruses, and respiratory syncytial virus (RSV) are the culprits behind viral illnesses. These viruses are frequently responsible for viral pneumonia and upper respiratory infections, such as the common cold. A common cause of flare-ups for long- term respiratory disorders including COPD and asthma is viral infections. Since antibiotics cannot treat viruses, supportive care—which includes rest, fluids, and over-the-counter drugs to ease symptoms—is the mainstay of treatment.

Understanding whether a respiratory infection is bacterial or viral is crucial for effective treatment, as misuse of antibiotics can lead to resistance and other complications.

Clinical Presentation: Fever, Productive Cough, Tachypnea

The clinical presentation of respiratory infections often includes fever, productive cough, and tachypnea, key indicators that help guide diagnosis and treatment.

One typical sign of respiratory infections is fever. It conveys the immune system's reaction to the illness. Sweating and chills may accompany it, indicating systemic involvement as the body attempts to combat the infection.

Productive cough is characterized by expulsing phlegm or mucus from the respiratory tract. The mucus may be yellow or green in bacterial infections, whereas viral infections might produce more apparent mucus. This symptom helps clear the airways of irritants and pathogens, but it can be persistent and exhausting.

Tachypnea, or rapid breathing, is observed when the body needs to increase oxygen intake to compensate for reduced lung function due to infection. This can be particularly distressing for patients, leading to feelings of breathlessness and fatigue.

These symptoms collectively contribute to the overall assessment and management of respiratory infections, guiding healthcare providers in their decisions regarding diagnostic testing and therapeutic interventions.

Diagnostic Tools: Chest X-ray, Sputum Culture

Healthcare providers often rely on diagnostic tools such as chest X-rays and sputum cultures to accurately diagnose respiratory infections and determine their severity.

Chest X-ray is a fundamental imaging tool that provides valuable insights into the condition of the lungs and airways. It can reveal signs of pneumonia, such as areas of opacity or lung consolidation, which indicate fluid or pus from the inflammatory response to the infection. Chest X-rays can also help detect other abnormalities, such as bronchitis, lung collapse, or pleural effusion, that might complicate the clinical picture.

Sputum culture is a microbiological test that examines mucus (sputum) coughed up from the respiratory tract in order to pinpoint the precise bacteria responsible for the infection. This test is beneficial for distinguishing between bacterial and viral infections and can help guide the choice of antibiotics in bacterial cases. Identifying the exact pathogen helps tailor treatment plans more effectively, ensuring appropriate medications that target the causative agent, optimizing recovery, and minimizing the risk of resistance.

Together, these diagnostic tools are crucial for confirming the presence of a respiratory infection, identifying its cause, and guiding appropriate treatment strategies.

Management: Antibiotics, Supportive Care (Oxygen, Fluids)

Effective management of respiratory infections typically involves a combination of antibiotics and supportive care measures.

Antibiotics are prescribed when the infection is determined to be bacterial. The choice of antibiotic depends on the specific pathogen identified through diagnostic tests like sputum culture, the patient's medical history, and local antibiotic resistance patterns. Timely administration is crucial to combat the infection and prevent complications, particularly in elderly patients or those with underlying health conditions.

Supportive care is vital in managing bacterial and viral respiratory infections. This includes administering oxygen therapy to patients experiencing significant breathing difficulties or low blood oxygen levels. Oxygen therapy helps ensure that vital organs receive adequate oxygen despite the lungs' compromised ability to absorb it. Drinking enough water is also important since it thins mucus discharges, making them simpler to evacuate and lowering the chance of further congestion. If the patient is unable to maintain oral intake, intravenous fluid administration may be necessary in more severe situations. Together, these therapeutic strategies help manage symptoms, support recovery and prevent the progression of respiratory infections.

Quick Clinical Assessment Checklist

A quick clinical assessment checklist for respiratory infections enables healthcare providers to efficiently diagnose and manage these conditions. Fever is an important evaluation parameter since it frequently represents the body's reaction to an illness. In addition, it's critical to evaluate the patient's breathing effort and rate, keeping an eye out for signs of respiratory distress such as tachypnea or the use of auxiliary muscles.

Evaluating the characteristics of a cough is necessary; noting whether it is dry or productive can help differentiate the type of infection and guide treatment decisions. Oxygen saturation should be measured using a pulse oximeter; low levels may require supplemental oxygen. Lastly, listening to lung sounds through auscultation can reveal wheezes, crackles, or decreased breath sounds, which provide further clues about the patient's respiratory status.

Respiratory Rate, Oxygen Saturation, Auscultation Findings

Critical assessments in evaluating respiratory infections include measuring the respiratory rate, checking oxygen saturation, and conducting a thorough auscultation. A higher-than-normal respiratory rate might be an indication of pneumonia or other dangerous diseases, or it could be the body's attempt to make up for low oxygen levels. Oxygen saturation, measured using a pulse oximeter, provides crucial information about gas exchange efficiency in the lungs. Values below 92% often require intervention, such as supplemental oxygen, to prevent organ damage.

Auscultation of the lungs can reveal abnormal sounds such as wheezing, crackles, or diminished breath sounds, suggesting different types of lung involvementtypes of lung involvement. Wheezing often points to airway narrowing or obstruction, crackles may indicate fluid in the air spaces, and diminished sounds suggest reduced airflow due to congestion or consolidation. These findings help refine the diagnosis, gauge the severity of the infection, and guide subsequent treatment decisions.

CHAPTER 3: ENDOCRINE SYSTEM

The endocrine system is a sophisticated network of glands that create and release hormones into the bloodstream, where they are subsequently transported to other organs. Numerous body processes are regulated by these hormones, such as development, metabolism, and mood. When these hormones' production or activity is disturbed, pathophysiology in the endocrine system ensues, giving rise to a range of illnesses.

Thyroid conditions, adrenal insufficiency, and diabetes mellitus are common endocrine illnesses. Diabetes results from insulin production or action issues, leading to abnormal glucose levels in the blood. Thyroid disorders, involving either overproduction (hyperthyroidism) or underproduction (hypothyroidism) of thyroid hormones, affect metabolism and energy levels. Adrenal insufficiency involves inadequate production of steroid hormones, which can affect metabolism, immune response, and stress responses.

Understanding the mechanisms behind these disruptions, such as autoimmune dysfunction, genetic factors, or environmental influences, is crucial for diagnosing, managing, and treating endocrine disorders. Restoring hormone balance and reducing symptoms are the goals of effective treatment, which enhances the quality of life for those who are impacted.

Key Hormonal Pathways
Important endocrine system hormonal pathways, especially those

involving thyroid and insulin hormones, are essential for preserving both general health and metabolic balance.

The beta cells in the pancreas create insulin, which is necessary for controlling blood glucose levels. It promotes the absorption of glucose by cells, encouraging its use as fuel and allowing the liver to store surplus glucose as glycogen. Diabetes mellitus can result from an inability to produce or use insulin. Insulin shortage is the outcome of beta cell death caused by the autoimmune system in type 1 diabetes. On the other hand, insulin resistance, which is frequently made worse by dietary and lifestyle choices, is a component of Type 2 diabetes.

Thyroxine (T4) and triiodothyronine (T3) are two of the thyroid hormones generated by the thyroid gland, which are essential for controlling growth, development, and metabolism. These hormones control heart rate, muscular strength, and metabolic rate, and they have an impact on nearly every organ system.

Imbalances in thyroid hormones can lead to hypothyroidism, characterized by insufficient hormone production, or hyperthyroidism, where excessive amounts are produced. Both conditions have significant physiological repercussions, affecting everything from energy levels to body temperature regulation.

Understanding and managing these hormonal pathways are pivotal in treating disorders that stem from their imbalance, ensuring proper metabolic function and overall health stability.

Critical Conditions and Management:

Critical conditions in the endocrine system include diabetes mellitus, thyroid disorders, and adrenal dysfunction, each requiring specific management strategies to maintain health and prevent complications.

The goal of managing diabetes mellitus is to keep blood glucose levels within a predetermined range. Medication, dietary adjustments, and lifestyle modifications can help achieve this. Whereas Type 2 diabetes may be controlled with oral hypoglycemics and occasionally insulin, Type 1 diabetes usually requires frequent insulin injections. It's also critical to teach people how to check their blood sugar levels.

Thyroid disorders require different approaches depending on whether the thyroid is overactive or underactive. Radiation therapy with iodine to diminish thyroid tissue or drugs that inhibit the synthesis of thyroid hormones are two possible treatments for hyperthyroidism. Hypothyroidism generally calls for hormone replacement therapy to supplement the necessary thyroid hormone the body lacks.

For adrenal dysfunction, such as Addison's disease, hormone replacement therapy is often necessary to correct hormone deficiencies. Conversely, conditions like Cushing's syndrome, characterized by excess cortisol, may require surgery, radiation, or medication to reduce cortisol production.

These management strategies are tailored to restore hormone balance and reduce symptoms, with regular follow-up and therapy adjustments critical to their effectiveness. This comprehensive approach helps improve patient outcomes and quality of life.

Diabetes Mellitus:

Diabetes mellitus is a metabolic disease marked by elevated blood glucose levels brought on by deficiencies in the generation or function of insulin. A complete lack of insulin results from the immune system of the body attacking and destroying the pancreatic beta cells that produce insulin in Type 1 diabetes. To control blood sugar levels in this disease, insulin treatment must be taken continuously.

The body either grows resistant to insulin or produces insufficient amounts to maintain normal glucose levels in those with Type 2 diabetes. The mainstays of care include weight control, frequent exercise, eating a balanced diet, and oral medicines. When blood sugar control with oral drugs is not achieved, insulin treatment may become essential.

Types: Gestational Diabetes

There are three main forms of diabetes mellitus: Type 1, Type 2, and gestational diabetes.

When the immune system unintentionally targets the pancreatic beta cells that produce insulin, type 1 diabetes results in a complete lack of insulin. Though it can occur at any age, it usually develops in childhood or adolescent. Blood glucose levels must be managed with lifetime insulin treatment in order to stay within a healthy range.

The most prevalent kind of diabetes, type 2, is caused by a loss in insulin production over time together with insulin resistance, a condition in which the body's cells do not respond to insulin as intended. Lifestyle issues including obesity, poor food, and inactivity are frequently associated with it. Oral drugs, lifestyle changes, and occasionally insulin are all part of management.

When hormonal changes during pregnancy cause insulin resistance, gestational diabetes develops. It normally disappears after delivery, but it raises the chance of acquiring Type 2 diabetes later in life. Management focuses on food, exercise, and occasionally insulin to regulate blood sugar levels and maintain a healthy pregnancy.

Pathophysiology

The two main pathophysiological factors of diabetes are beta-cell

49

malfunction and insulin resistance. Insulin resistance is a condition in which the body's cells, especially those in the muscles, fat, and liver, do not react to insulin as they should. This resistance hinders glucose uptake by the cells, causing glucose to remain in the bloodstream. The pancreas produces more insulin to compensate, but this effort becomes inadequate over time, leading to elevated blood sugar levels.

The reduced capacity of the pancreatic beta cells to generate and release insulin is known as beta-cell dysfunction. In Type 2 diabetes, chronic insulin resistance places excessive demand on these cells, causing them to deteriorate and produce less insulin. One feature of diabetes is chronic hyperglycemia, which is brought on by a combination of insulin resistance and decreased insulin production. Understanding these mechanisms is crucial for targeted management strategies, improving insulin sensitivity, and supporting beta-cell function.

Clinical Features: Polyuria, Polydipsia, Weight Loss

Diabetes mellitus presents with vital clinical features, including polyuria, polydipsia, and weight loss.

Polyuria, or frequent urination, is caused by an excess of glucose in the blood that seeps into the urine and draws water with it. This increased urination starts a vicious cycle of fluid loss and dehydration.

Polydipsia results from this dehydration. As the body loses fluids through frequent urination, excessive thirst triggers to compensate for the water loss, causing individuals to drink more fluids.

When insulin, which is required for glucose utilization, is absent from the body, weight loss occurs, especially in untreated Type 1 diabetes, as the body begins to break down fat and muscle for energy. These symptoms often signal the presence of diabetes and prompt further investigation.

Diagnostic Criteria: Fasting Glucose, HbA1c, OGTT

Specific criteria, such as fasting blood glucose levels, HbA1c values, and the oral glucose tolerance test (OGTT), are used to diagnose diabetes mellitus.

Blood sugar levels are measured using fasting glucose following a minimum eight-hour overnight fast. Diabetes is indicated by two fasting blood glucose readings of 126 mg/dL (7.0 mmol/L) or above.

The average blood glucose levels over the previous two to three months are reflected in the HbA1c. Diabetes can be diagnosed with a HbA1c result of 6.5% or above. This test is beneficial since it offers a more extended perspective on blood sugar regulation.

Two hours after ingesting a drink high in glucose, blood glucose is measured as part of the OGTT protocol. Diabetes is confirmed by a blood glucose level at the two-hour mark of 200 mg/dL (11.1

mmol/L) or above. This test determines the efficiency of the body's glucose metabolism.

Management

The goal of diabetes management is to keep blood glucose levels within a healthy range by controlling food, using insulin, and using oral hypoglycemics.

When other therapies are not enough, insulin therapy is necessary for people with Type 1 diabetes and occasionally for those with Type 2 diabetes. In order to control blood sugar, insulin is given by injections or an insulin pump, imitating the body's normal release of insulin.

The main goals of oral hypoglycemics in the treatment of Type 2 diabetes are to increase insulin sensitivity, increase insulin production, or reduce the absorption of glucose. Metformin, which enhances the body's reaction to insulin, and sulfonylureas, which increase the synthesis of insulin, are examples of common drugs.

One of the most important aspects of controlling any kind of diabetes is diet control. A well- balanced diet that is low in fiber and processed carbohydrates aids in blood sugar stabilization. Blood glucose spikes may be avoided by keeping an eye on carbohydrate consumption and selecting foods with a low glycemic index, which will aid in overall control efforts.

Thyroid Disorders (Hyperthyroidism, Hypothyroidism):

Thyroid disorders, including hyperthyroidism and hypothyroidism, result from imbalances in thyroid hormone production, impacting metabolism and overall bodily function.

An increased metabolism results from the thyroid gland producing too much thyroid hormone (T3 and T4), a condition known as hyperthyroidism. Sweating, an increased hunger, nervousness, weight loss, and a fast pulse are typical symptoms. Thyroiditis, toxic nodular goiter, and Graves' disease are the most frequent causes. Treatment options include radioactive iodine treatment, antithyroid drugs, and, in extreme situations, surgery to stop hormone production.

The hallmark of hypothyroidism is inadequate thyroid hormone synthesis, which slows down metabolic functions. Fatigue, weight gain, cold intolerance, dry skin, and sadness are some of the symptoms. The most frequent cause is an autoimmune condition called Hashimoto's thyroiditis, in which the thyroid gland is attacked by the immune system. In order to regulate hormone levels and reduce symptoms, daily thyroid hormone replacement therapy—typically with levothyroxine—is the standard of care.

Pathophysiology: Autoimmunity, Iodine Deficiency

The pathophysiology of thyroid disorders often involves

autoimmunity and iodine deficiency.

Under autoimmune diseases, the thyroid gland is erroneously attacked by the body's immune system. Conditions such as Graves' disease induce the immune system to create antibodies, which in turn drive the thyroid to release excess hormones, leading to hyperthyroidism. Conversely, in hypothyroidism, Hashimoto's thyroiditis leads to immune cells attacking the thyroid tissue, impairing its ability to produce hormones, resulting in an underactive thyroid.

Iodine deficiency plays a key role, especially in hypothyroidism. Iodine is essential for synthesizing thyroid hormones, and a deficiency reduces the gland's ability to produce adequate hormones, causing metabolic slowing. This deficiency can also lead to goiter, an enlargement of the thyroid as it attempts to compensate for the lack of hormone production. It is essential to comprehend these mechanisms in order to diagnose and treat thyroid diseases.

Clinical Features: Weight Changes, Heat/Cold Intolerance, Fatigue

Thyroid disorders present with distinct clinical features, often reflecting the body's altered metabolic state.

Weight changes are expected. In hyperthyroidism, an overactive thyroid accelerates metabolism, leading to unintentional weight loss despite an increased appetite. In contrast, hypothyroidism slows metabolism, often resulting in weight gain, even with a standard or reduced diet.

Another key symptom is heat or cold intolerance. Hyperthyroid patients often experience heat intolerance, feeling excessively warm and sweating quickly. Those with hypothyroidism typically have cold intolerance, frequently feeling chilled and having difficulty staying warm.

Fatigue is prevalent in both conditions. Hyperthyroidism can cause muscle weakness and exhaustion due to an overactive metabolic state. Hypothyroidism leads to tiredness and sluggishness as the body's slowed processes drain energy. Recognizing these features aids in early diagnosis and effective management.

Diagnostics: TSH, Free T4, Thyroid Ultrasound

Imaging and blood testing are used in tandem to diagnose thyroid problems. The principal test for assessing thyroid function is the TSH (thyroid-stimulating hormone) test. TSH levels are raised in hypothyroidism as a result of the body's attempt to encourage an underactive thyroid to generate more hormones. On the other hand, TSH levels are usually low in hyperthyroidism because the pituitary gland's TSH release is suppressed by the overproduction of thyroid hormones.

Free T4 (Thyroxine) measures the unbound, active form of the thyroid hormone in the blood. Elevated free T4 levels indicate hyperthyroidism, while decreased levels suggest hypothyroidism. This test provides a clearer picture of the thyroid's activity, especially when abnormal TSH results.

Thyroid ultrasound visualizes the thyroid gland's structure. It helps identify abnormalities like nodules, enlargement, or inflammation, which can be associated with goiter, Graves' disease, or Hashimoto's thyroiditis. Together, these diagnostic tools provide a comprehensive assessment of thyroid health and guide appropriate treatment.

Management

Management of thyroid disorders depends on whether the condition is hypothyroidism or hyperthyroidism.

Levothyroxine, a synthetic version of the thyroid hormone thyroxine, is the main medication used to treat hypothyroidism (T4). This drug is used on a regular basis to relieve symptoms such as weariness, weight gain, and cold sensitivity, as well as to return hormone levels to normal. To guarantee ideal dose, TSH and free T4 levels are often checked and the dosage is adjusted according on the patient's demands.

Methimazole is frequently used to lessen the overproduction of thyroid hormones in cases of hyperthyroidism. Methimazole helps manage symptoms including weight loss, heat intolerance, and a fast heartbeat by preventing the thyroid gland from producing hormones. Radioactive iodine therapy is an additional treatment option for hyperthyroidism that entails ingesting a dosage of radioactive iodine that specifically eliminates hyperactive thyroid tissue. Thyroid hormone levels are frequently gradually reduced as a result of this medication, which might occasionally necessitate lifetime thyroid hormone replacement.

These treatments aim to stabilize thyroid function, relieve symptoms, and prevent complications, improving overall quality of life for individuals with thyroid disorders.

Quick Clinical Assessment Checklist

A quick clinical assessment checklist for thyroid disorders includes evaluating key symptoms, physical examination findings, and initial diagnostic tests.

Start by inquiring about typical symptoms including changes in appetite, weariness, heat or cold intolerance, unexplained weight fluctuations, heart palpitations, and any recent mood swings like worry or sadness. Keep an eye on the patient's energy levels and take note of any indicators of fatigue or restlessness.

Perform a physical examination focusing on the neck to check for thyroid enlargement, nodules, or tenderness. Along with assessing heart rate and rhythm, one should search for indications of bradycardia in hypothyroidism or tachycardia in hyperthyroidism. Check for signs like dry skin, hair loss, and reflex changes, indicating hormonal imbalances.

Conclude with initial diagnostic tests, including TSH and free T4 levels, to identify thyroid dysfunction. This quick assessment guides the next steps in confirming a diagnosis and determining the appropriate management plan.

Blood Glucose Monitoring, Symptom Review for Endocrine Disorders

Blood glucose monitoring and symptom review are essential in managing endocrine disorders like diabetes and thyroid dysfunction.

It is essential for diabetic people to check their blood sugar levels using blood glucose monitoring. Frequent monitoring aids in regulating food consumption, exercise, and medication to keep blood glucose levels within the desired range. In order to monitor their daily levels throughout fasting, pre-meal, and post-meal times, patients frequently utilize glucometers. Real-time data from continuous glucose monitoring (CGM) devices helps with better decision- making by providing a more complete picture of glucose swings.

Symptom review plays a vital role in assessing overall endocrine health. Patients should report symptoms such as unexplained weight changes, excessive thirst, frequent urination, fatigue, temperature intolerance, mood alterations, or changes in appetite. These symptoms can signal changes in blood glucose control or thyroid hormone imbalances. Regular symptom review guides healthcare providers in adjusting treatment plans to prevent complications and improve patient outcomes.

CHAPTER 4:
GASTROINTESTINAL
SYSTEM

The digestive tract (GI) is in charge of breaking down food, taking in nutrients, and eliminating waste. Pathophysiology in this system develops from abnormalities in normal function, which can result in a number of diseases, including GERD, IBS, and inflammatory bowel disease (IBD). These conditions may be brought on by infection, inflammation, autoimmune, or lifestyle decisions. Abdominal discomfort, bloating, diarrhea, constipation, and nausea are typical symptoms. Effective management often involves dietary adjustments, medications to reduce inflammation or acid production, and lifestyle changes to improve digestion and overall gut health, tailored to the specific GI condition.

Gastrointestinal Pathophysiology

Gastrointestinal pathophysiology involves:

- Deviations from the digestive system's regular course.
- Affecting processes like digestion.
- Nutrient absorption.
- Waste elimination.

Various factors contribute to these disorders, including inflammation, infection, autoimmune responses, structural abnormalities, and lifestyle influences such as diet and stress.

The GI tract is chronically inflamed in conditions such as inflammatory bowel disease (IBD). In contrast, gastroesophageal reflux disease (GERD) results from acid backflow into the esophagus due to a weakened lower esophageal sphincter. Changes in bowel habits and abdominal discomfort are the hallmarks of irritable bowel syndrome (IBS), which is frequently brought on by food and stress factors. Understanding these underlying mechanisms is crucial for accurate diagnosis and effective management.

Functional Anatomy of the GI Tract

From the mouth to the anus, the gastrointestinal (GI) tract is a continuous, hollow tube. The mouth, esophagus, stomach, small intestine, large intestine, and rectum are among its main parts. Every component has a distinct role in nutrition absorption and digestion.

The mouth starts the digestive process, breaking down food with saliva and chewing. Peristalsis is the term for the rhythmic contractions that the esophagus uses to transfer food to the stomach. Food is broken down by stomach acids and enzymes in the gut, becoming a semi- liquid chyme. The primary location of nutritional absorption is the small intestine, which includes the ileum, jejunum, and duodenum. Here, nutrients are further broken down by bile from the liver and digestive enzymes from the pancreas. Solid waste is formed in the large intestine by the absorption of water and electrolytes. Lastly, waste products are held in the rectum until they are released through the anus. It takes this concerted effort to sustain general health.

Critical Conditions and Management:

Several vital conditions can affect the gastrointestinal (GI) tract, each requiring specific management strategies to alleviate symptoms and prevent complications.

The GI tract is chronically inflamed in inflammatory bowel diseases (IBD), such as Crohn's disease and ulcerative colitis. The goal of management is to control symptoms and lower inflammation by using drugs such as biologics, corticosteroids, aminosalicylates, and immunomodulators. It may also be required to make dietary changes and, in certain situations, undergo surgery.

Heartburn and discomfort are brought on by stomach acid refluxing back into the esophagus, a condition known as gastroesophageal reflux disease (GERD). Lifestyle modifications including avoiding trigger foods, sleeping with your head up, and controlling your weight are all part of treatment. While antacids offer immediate relief, medications such as proton pump inhibitors (PPIs) and H2 blockers aid in reducing the generation of acid.

The symptoms of Irritable Bowel Syndrome (IBS), a functional illness, include bloating, altered bowel habits, and abdominal discomfort. Dietary changes include consuming more fiber, avoiding trigger foods, and managing stress as part of the treatment. Medication such as laxatives, antispasmodics, or antidiarrheal drugs may also be utilized, depending on the symptoms.

Tailoring management to the specific GI condition improves patient comfort and overall health outcomes.

Inflammatory Bowel Diseases (Crohn's, Ulcerative Colitis):

The term "inflammatory bowel diseases" (IBD) refers to a group of illnesses that include ulcerative colitis and Crohn's disease, both of which are marked by persistent gastrointestinal tract inflammation.

Any area of the gastrointestinal system, from the mouth to the anus, can be impacted by Crohn's disease, which frequently affects the intestine wall's deeper layers. Abdominal discomfort, diarrhea, exhaustion, weight loss, and occasionally fever are among the symptoms.

Because it is uneven, there may be spaces of healthy tissue in between inflammatory segments, which can result in problems like strictures or fistulas.

The colon and rectum are the main organs affected by ulcerative colitis, which results in inflammation and ulcers in the innermost lining. Symptoms include bloody diarrhea, urgency, abdominal cramping, and weight loss. Unlike Crohn's, ulcerative colitis presents as a continuous area of inflammation.

The goals of IBD management are to keep the disease in remission, reduce inflammation, and manage symptoms. Commonly used medications include corticosteroids, immunomodulators, biologics, and aminosalicylates. In severe situations, intestinal damage may need to be removed surgically. In addition to diet, lifestyle changes—including stress reduction—are essential for controlling chronic illnesses and enhancing quality of life.

Pathophysiology

The pathophysiology of Inflammatory Bowel Disease (IBD), which encompasses Crohn's disease and ulcerative colitis, is primarily focused on immune-mediated inflammation. In both conditions, the immune system mistakenly identifies components of the gastrointestinal tract as harmful, triggering a chronic inflammatory response.

The immune system and the gut bacteria interact abnormally, which triggers the start of this process. The control of the immune system in the gut can be disturbed by both genetic and environmental influences. T-cells and other immune cells are activated in response, releasing inflammatory cytokines such interleukins and TNF-alpha. The gut lining becomes damaged as a result of these cytokines' promotion of continuous inflammation.

This inflammation can spread throughout the GI tract in patches and permeate all layers of the gut wall in cases of Crohn's disease. Usually, ulcerative colitis only affects the mucosal layer of the colon and the rectum. Symptoms include diarrhea, bleeding, and stomach discomfort are brought on by this immune-mediated onslaught, which interferes with normal gut function. In addition, it may result in problems including fistulas, strictures, or a higher chance of colon cancer. Comprehending this immune-stimulated inflammation is essential for directing anti- inflammatory and immunosuppressive drug therapy.

Clinical Features

Consisting of diarrhea, bleeding in the rectal area, and discomfort in the stomach, these are the clinical signs of Crohn's disease, ulcerative colitis, and other inflammatory bowel disorders (IBD).

Abdominal pain is a common symptom that often results from inflammation and ulceration of the intestinal lining. While Crohn's illness can cause abdominal pain anywhere, ulcerative colitis often affects the lower left side.

Diarrhea is frequent, often urgent, and can range from mild to severe. Due to inflammation and ulceration of the colon lining, diarrhea in Crohn's disease is often watery, but in ulcerative colitis, it may also be accompanied with mucus and blood.

Rectal bleeding is more common in ulcerative colitis but can also occur in Crohn's disease, especially when the colon is involved. The blood results from ulcers and erosions in the intestinal lining, indicating active inflammation. These clinical features are crucial in suspecting and diagnosing IBD, guiding further investigation and treatment.

Diagnostic Tools

Diagnostic Tools for Inflammatory Bowel Diseases (IBD) include colonoscopy, CRP (C-reactive protein) levels, and fecal calprotectin.

A colonoscopy is the most definitive diagnostic tool. It allows direct visualization of the intestinal lining and identifies inflammation, ulceration, and bleeding. Biopsies gathered during the operation can distinguish Crohn's disease from ulcerative colitis based on tissue features.

C-reactive protein, or CRP, is a blood test used to gauge an individual's level of inflammation. Elevated CRP levels suggest active inflammation in IBD, though they are not specific and can also be elevated in other conditions.

The presence of calprotectin, a protein secreted by white blood cells during inflammation, may be determined using a non-invasive stool test called fecal calprotectin. Raised levels can be used to differentiate IBD from non-inflammatory diseases such as irritable bowel syndrome (IBS) since they signify ongoing intestinal inflammation.

Management

Management of IBD focuses on reducing inflammation, controlling symptoms, and maintaining remission.

Aminosalicylates, such as mesalamine, are often used in mild to moderate ulcerative colitis to reduce inflammation in the intestinal lining.

Immunomodulators like azathioprine and methotrexate suppress the immune system to prevent ongoing inflammation and help maintain long-term remission.

Biologics (e.g., infliximab, adalimumab) are used for moderate to severe IBD. They target specific immune response components, such as TNF-alpha, to control inflammation more effectively and promote healing of the intestinal lining.

With the goal of enhancing the patient's quality of life, these treatment techniques are customized based on the kind and severity of the illness.

Gastroesophageal Reflux Disease (GERD):

The disorder known as gastroesophageal reflux disease (GERD) is characterized by the regurgitation of stomach acid into the esophagus, irritating its lining.

Pathophysiology: Lower Esophageal Sphincter Dysfunction

The lower esophageal sphincter (LES), a ring of muscle at the opening between the esophagus and stomach, is dysfunctional, and this is part of the pathogenesis. The LES typically serves as a barrier, opening to let food enter the stomach and shutting to stop reflux of stomach contents. The LES weakens or relaxes abnormally in GERD, which permits acidic stomach contents to reflux back into the esophagus. The esophageal lining becomes irritated and inflamed as a result of reflux, giving rise to the typical GERD symptoms.

Clinical Features: Heartburn, Regurgitation

The two main clinical characteristics are regurgitation and heartburn. A burning feeling in the chest, heartburn frequently gets worse after eating or sleeping. It happens when the esophagus becomes irritated by the stomach's acidic contents. Regurgitation is the process by which food or sour liquid from the stomach flows backward into the mouth or throat, leaving behind an unpleasant taste.

These symptoms can significantly impact daily life, leading to discomfort, disrupted sleep, and, if left untreated, complications such as esophagitis or Barrett's esophagus.

Diagnostics: Endoscopy, pH Monitoring

Gastroesophageal Reflux Disease (GERD) Diagnostics primarily include endoscopy and pH monitoring.

During an endoscopy, the esophagus is visually inspected for indications of inflammation, ulcers, or other damage brought on by acid reflux. An endoscope, or flexible tube containing a camera, is inserted down the throat during this treatment to give a clear image of the esophagus lining. In order to rule out other disorders, such Barrett's esophagus, biopsies can also be performed.

Over the course of a day, pH monitoring gauges the acidity of the esophagus. An esophageal tiny probe is inserted to measure the frequency and length of acid reflux episodes. This test, particularly in cases when the diagnosis is unclear, aids in the confirmation of GERD and evaluates the degree of acid exposure.

Management: PPIs, H2 Blockers, Lifestyle Modifications

Management of GERD focuses on reducing acid production and improving lifestyle factors to prevent reflux.

Omeprazole and esomeprazole are two examples of proton pump inhibitors (PPIs), which are the best drugs for decreasing the production of stomach acid. They relieve symptoms and encourage the lining of the esophagus to mend.

H2 blockers, like ranitidine and famotidine, decrease stomach acid production. They are less potent than PPIs but can be helpful for mild to moderate symptoms.

Lifestyle modifications play a crucial role in managing GERD. These include avoiding trigger foods (e.g., spicy foods, caffeine, chocolate), eating smaller meals, not lying down immediately after eating, elevating the head during sleep, and maintaining a healthy weight. These combined strategies help control symptoms, improve quality of life, and prevent complications.

Quick Clinical Assessment Checklist

A quick clinical assessment for gastrointestinal (GI) conditions includes a thorough abdominal examination and the identification of red flags for potential GI bleeding.

Abdominal Examination, Red Flags for GI Bleeding

The abdominal examination involves inspecting, palpating, and auscultating the abdomen. Look for any visible signs like distension, surgical scars, or abnormal movements. Palpate gently to assess for tenderness, masses, or organ enlargement. There may be localized tenderness or guarding in cases of inflammation or obstruction. Auscultation helps identify changes in bowel sounds, with hypoactive sounds suggesting obstruction or ileus and hyperactive sounds pointing to irritation or early obstruction.

Hematemesis (blood in the vomit), melena (black, tarry stools), and hematochezia (bright red blood in the stool) are examples of

70

symptoms that indicate gastrointestinal bleeding. Diaphoresis, prolonged exhaustion, and unexplained anemia are other alarming symptoms that point to possible chronic blood loss. In order to identify the cause and extent of the bleeding and to establish the best course of action, these symptoms need to be looked at very away. Early detection of these symptoms can guarantee prompt intervention and avoid problems.

CHAPTER 5: RENAL SYSTEM

The renal system filters blood, eliminates waste, and controls fluid and electrolyte levels—all of which are essential for preserving the body's internal equilibrium. The main organs of this system, the kidneys, also regulate blood pressure, balance pH, create urine, and release hormones that affect the creation of red blood cells. These processes can be severely disrupted by pathophysiological alterations in the renal system, which can result in electrolyte imbalances, acute renal damage, and chronic kidney disease. It is essential to comprehend the intricate workings and anatomical structure of the renal system in order to diagnose and treat a variety of kidney-related conditions.

Renal Function and Homeostasis

The field of renal pathophysiology is concerned with the effects of kidney dysfunction on the body's capacity to sustain homeostasis. The kidneys control water, electrolyte balance, acid-base balance, and blood filtration in addition to eliminating waste. Electrolyte abnormalities, chronic renal disease, and acute kidney damage can result from impairments in these functions.

The kidneys use a number of mechanisms to keep the body in equilibrium. Urine is released after they filter blood, removing waste materials including creatinine and urea. They also maintain appropriate hydration by controlling water absorption, which controls fluid levels. Through selective filtration and reabsorption, electrolytes like salt, potassium, and calcium are balanced, which has a direct impact on nerve function and blood pressure. The kidneys' excretion of hydrogen ions and absorption of bicarbonate contribute to the maintenance of the acid-base balance.

Another essential component of kidney function is the generation of hormones, such as erythropoietin for the formation of red blood cells and renin for the regulation of blood pressure. Renal pathophysiology is important to understand since disruptions to these systems can result in serious health problems.

Critical Conditions and Management:

Chronic Kidney Disease (CKD) is a progressive condition where the kidneys lose their ability to filter blood effectively. Management focuses on slowing progression through blood pressure control, often using ACE inhibitors or ARBs, and maintaining blood sugar levels in diabetic patients. Dietary modifications, such as reducing sodium, protein, and phosphorus intake, help manage symptoms and prevent complications. Advanced stages may require dialysis or kidney transplantation.

An abrupt reduction in kidney function is known as acute kidney injury (AKI), and it is frequently brought on by toxic medication exposure, infections, or dehydration. Management consists of:

- Identifying and treating the underlying cause.
- Restoring fluid balance.
- Avoiding medications that may worsen kidney function.

Temporary dialysis may be required in extreme situations to maintain renal function while the patient recovers.

Electrolyte Imbalances are common in renal conditions. Management involves carefully monitoring electrolyte levels, such as sodium, potassium, and calcium, and adjusting diet or medications to correct imbalances. For example, high potassium levels (hyperkalemia) may require dietary restrictions, drugs, or dialysis to prevent life-threatening complications.

In order to maximize kidney health, effective therapy of many renal diseases necessitates regular monitoring, lifestyle modifications, and patient-provider teamwork.

Chronic Kidney Disease (CKD):

The gradual decrease of kidney function over months or years is known as chronic kidney disease (CKD). It occurs when the kidneys are damaged and cannot filter blood efficiently, accumulating waste products and fluid imbalances in the body. Common causes include diabetes, hypertension, glomerulonephritis, and prolonged use of nephrotoxic medications.

Early stages of CKD are often asymptomatic, but as it advances, symptoms like fatigue, swelling (edema), high blood pressure, and changes in urine output may develop. Management focuses on slowing disease progression through blood pressure control with medications such as ACE inhibitors or ARBs, blood sugar management in diabetic patients, and dietary changes. Dialysis or kidney transplantation may be used as treatments in later stages to restore lost kidney function. For CKD to be adequately managed, monitoring renal function, electrolyte levels, and general health is essential.

Stages: GFR Categories, Albuminuria

Based on the presence of albuminuria, which indicates the degree of kidney damage and function, and the glomerular filtration rate (GFR), Chronic Kidney Disease (CKD) is categorized into phases.

GFR Categories help indicate the severity of kidney dysfunction. There are five stages:

- Stage 1: Normal kidney function with a GFR of at least 90 mL/min/1.73 m^ �, but signs of kidney damage, such as protein in the urine.
- Stage 2: GFR 60-89, which represents a moderate decline in renal function.
- Stage 3: GFR 30-59, which denotes the start of discernible symptoms and significant renal impairment.
- Stage 4: GFR 15–29, which indicates a severe decline in renal function and is frequently accompanied by symptoms such as weariness, edema, and altered urine patterns.
- Stage 5: GFR < 15, which indicates end-stage renal illness and necessitates dialysis or kidney transplantation.

Albuminuria is the term used to describe the presence of albumin, a sign of kidney impairment, in the urine. A1 (normal to mildly raised), A2 (moderately increased), and A3 (severely increased) are the three categories into which it is divided. Increased likelihood of disease development and more substantial kidney injury are indicated by increased albuminuria levels. For determining the severity of CKD, directing treatment, and forecasting results, GFR and albuminuria are essential.

Pathophysiology: Nephron Loss, Compensatory Hyperfiltration

Chronic Kidney Disease (CKD) pathophysiology primarily involves the progressive loss of nephrons and compensatory hyperfiltration. The kidney's functional components, called nephrons, are in charge of filtering blood and preserving electrolyte and fluid balance. In CKD, various factors, such as diabetes, hypertension, or glomerulonephritis, lead to the gradual destruction of nephrons.

As nephrons are lost, the remaining functional nephrons undergo compensatory hyperfiltration to maintain overall kidney function. This means the surviving nephrons work harder, increasing their filtration rate to compensate for the loss. Initially, this adaptation helps preserve kidney function, but over time, the increased workload further damages these remaining nephrons. This damage results in glomerular hypertension, increased permeability, and proteinuria, which further accelerates the progression of CKD. This cycle of nephron loss and hyperfiltration continues, eventually leading to a decline in overall kidney function.

Clinical Features: Anemia, Electrolyte Imbalance, Edema

Chronic Kidney Disease (CKD) presents with several clinical features, including anemia, electrolyte imbalances, and edema.

When the kidneys are unable to generate enough erythropoietin—a hormone that promotes the creation of red blood cells—anemia sets in. Weakness, exhaustion, and pallor are indications of decreased erythropoietin levels, which lead to a decrease in red blood cells.

Electrolyte imbalances are common in CKD. The kidneys struggle to regulate essential electrolytes, leading to elevated potassium (hyperkalemia), which can affect heart function, and decreased calcium, which weakens bones. Phosphorus levels also often rise, contributing to bone disease and calcium imbalance.

The inability of the kidneys to eliminate extra fluid leads to edema. Swelling results from this fluid retention, especially in the legs, ankles, and eye area. Edema is a sign of declining renal function and has to be carefully managed to avoid consequences like heart failure. It is essential to identify these characteristics in order to diagnose CKD and develop effective treatment plans.

Diagnostics: Serum Creatinine, eGFR, Urinalysis

A urinalysis, the estimated glomerular filtration rate (eGFR), and serum creatinine levels are three crucial tests in the diagnosis of chronic kidney disease (CKD).

Serum creatinine is a blood test that quantifies the level of creatinine, a waste product of muscle metabolism that is typically eliminated by the kidneys. Since the kidneys are less efficient in removing this waste, an elevated blood creatinine level is indicative of decreased renal function.

To determine the kidneys' capability for filtering blood, eGFR is computed using serum creatinine, age, sex, and body size information. It gives a general picture of renal function and aids in CKD stage classification, directing management and therapy choices.

Urinalysis involves examining urine for abnormalities such as protein (proteinuria) or blood (hematuria). Protein, mainly albumin, suggests kidney damage and is a marker of CKD progression. Detecting abnormalities in urinalysis is crucial for early diagnosis and ongoing monitoring of kidney health. Together, these tests provide a comprehensive assessment of kidney function and damage, informing treatment strategies.

Management: ACE Inhibitors, Dialysis, Nutritional Modifications

In order to control symptoms and reduce the disease's course, chronic kidney disease (CKD) management strategies include medication, lifestyle modifications, and, in more advanced stages, medical procedures.

ACE inhibitors are frequently used to CKD patients in order to control excessive blood pressure and lessen proteinuria. They function by decreasing blood pressure, loosening blood arteries, and lessening renal strain. This aids in preventing additional kidney damage, especially in those with renal disease brought on by diabetes or hypertension.

Dialysis becomes necessary in advanced stages of CKD (stage 5) when kidney function declines significantly. It performs the filtering tasks of the kidneys by removing waste products and excess fluids and balancing electrolytes. Hemodialysis, which filters blood using a machine, and peritoneal dialysis, which utilizes the lining of the belly to remove waste materials, are the two primary forms.

Making dietary changes is essential for controlling CKD. Patients are frequently instructed to restrict their consumption of sodium, potassium, and phosphorus in order to avoid electrolyte abnormalities.

Protein intake may also be moderated to reduce the kidneys' workload. Fluid intake might be regulated based on the kidney function level and symptoms like edema. These dietary adjustments help maintain balance and prevent complications associated with CKD.

Acute Kidney Injury (AKI):

Acute Kidney Injury (AKI) is a rapid loss of kidney function that can happen in a matter of hours or days. As a result, the kidneys are unable to control acid-base status, preserve fluid and electrolyte balance, and filter waste products. Dehydration, serious infections, medication toxicity (including NSAIDs and some antibiotics), and illnesses like heart failure that lower blood flow to the kidneys are common causes of AKI.

AKI can cause mild to severe symptoms, such as decreased urine production, ankle and leg edema, exhaustion, disorientation, and nausea. Early recognition and intervention are critical in AKI, as prompt treatment can often reverse kidney damage. Management focuses on identifying and treating the underlying cause, restoring fluid balance, adjusting medications that may impact kidney function, and providing supportive care. In severe cases, temporary dialysis may be required to support kidney function until recovery occurs.

Types: Pre-renal, Intrinsic, Post-renal

Based on the underlying etiology, acute kidney injury (AKI) is divided into three categories: pre-renal, intrinsic, and post-renal.

Reduced blood supply to the kidneys, frequently as a result of dehydration, heart failure, or substantial blood loss, is the cause of pre-renal AKI. The kidneys are initially healthy, but a lack of blood supply reduces their ability to filter waste. If not addressed quickly, it can progress to intrinsic damage.

Intrinsic AKI directly damages the kidneys, affecting the nephrons and other structures. Common causes include acute tubular necrosis (from toxins or ischemia), glomerulonephritis, and interstitial nephritis. This type of AKI requires identifying the specific injury to guide appropriate treatment.

Urine flow restriction in the urinary system, such as kidney stones, tumors, or an enlarged prostate, can result in post-renal acute kidney injury (AKI). This blockage causes pressure to build up in the kidneys, reducing their filtering capacity. If managed promptly, removing the obstruction often leads to recovery of kidney function.

Pathophysiology: Rapid Decline in Renal Function

The pathophysiology of acute kidney injury (AKI) involves a sudden decrease in renal function, which makes it more difficult for the kidneys to balance fluids, filter waste, and control electrolytes. This decline can occur within hours to days and results from various underlying causes.

Reduced blood flow to the kidneys causes inadequate oxygen and nutrition delivery, which compromises the kidneys' ability to filter. This is known as pre-renal AKI. This decreased perfusion has the potential to harm renal tissue and result in intrinsic injury if it persists.

Intrinsic AKI involves direct damage to the kidney structures, such as the tubules, glomeruli, or interstitium. This damage disrupts standard filtration and reabsorption processes, causing waste products like urea and creatinine to accumulate in the bloodstream.

Post-renal AKI occurs when a blockage in the urinary tract creates back pressure in the kidneys, interfering with their ability to filter blood. This obstruction hinders urine flow, leading to swelling and injury to kidney tissues.

All things considered, the rapid loss of kidney function associated with AKI causes fluid retention, electrolyte abnormalities (such as hyperkalemia), and metabolic acidosis, all of which can be fatal if left untreated.

Clinical Features: Oliguria, Elevated BUN/Creatinine

Important clinical signs of acute kidney injury (AKI) include oliguria, increased blood urea nitrogen (BUN), and high creatinine levels.

AKI is characterized by oligouria, which is defined as a substantial decrease in urine production (less than 400 mL per day in adults). It suggests that the kidneys are having difficulty producing urine and filtering blood. Fluid retention brought on by oligouria frequently manifests as symptoms such as edema in the ankles, legs, and eye area.

Elevated BUN and creatinine levels are critical indicators of AKI. BUN and creatinine are waste products filtered by healthy kidneys; an increase in these levels reflects the kidneys' reduced filtering ability. Elevated creatinine is significant for assessing the severity of AKI, while BUN can also provide insights into hydration status and protein metabolism. Monitoring these levels is essential for diagnosing AKI and guiding its management.

Management: Fluid Management, Electrolyte Correction

The primary goals of managing acute kidney injury (AKI) are to stabilize renal function and stop more damage from occurring. This is accomplished mainly by maintaining proper fluid and electrolyte balance.

Fluid management is crucial, as it addresses both dehydration and fluid overload. In cases of pre-renal AKI caused by dehydration or low blood volume, careful administration of intravenous fluids can restore blood flow to the kidneys and improve their filtering ability. Conversely, if fluid overload is present (evidenced by swelling and shortness of breath), diuretics may remove excess fluid and relieve pressure on the heart and kidneys.

Electrolyte correction involves monitoring and adjusting critical electrolyte levels, such as potassium, sodium, and calcium. Elevated potassium (hyperkalemia) is particularly dangerous, as it can cause life-threatening cardiac arrhythmias. Treatments may include dietary restrictions, medications to promote potassium excretion (such as diuretics), or emergency interventions like calcium gluconate or dialysis to reduce potassium levels rapidly. Correcting imbalances in sodium and calcium is also essential to maintain overall metabolic stability and prevent complications.

By managing fluid status and correcting electrolyte disturbances, the kidneys are supported in their recovery, reducing the risk of long-term damage.

Quick Clinical Assessment Checklist

A quick clinical assessment for Acute Kidney Injury (AKI) should include monitoring urine output, evaluating fluid status, and conducting regular electrolyte checks.

Urine Output, Fluid Status, Electrolyte Monitoring

Assess urine output by measuring the volume over a set period, as a drop in the production (oliguria) is often an early sign of AKI. Documenting any changes can help gauge kidney function and the effectiveness of interventions.

Evaluate fluid status by examining for signs of dehydration (dry mucous membranes, low blood pressure) or fluid overload (leg swelling, increased blood pressure, shortness of breath). This will guide decisions on fluid management, such as whether fluids need to be administered or restricted.

Conduct electrolyte monitoring, especially checking potassium, sodium, and calcium levels. Regular tests are vital to identify imbalances, such as hyperkalemia, that require immediate correction to prevent complications.

CHAPTER 6: NERVOUS SYSTEM

The nervous system is an intricate network that controls many body activities, including movement, thought, perception of sensory information, and autonomic responses. Disturbances in the regular operation of the nervous system are referred to as neurological pathophysiology. These can be caused by a number of things, including trauma, infections, genetic disorders, vascular problems, and degenerative illnesses.

The brain, spinal cord, and peripheral nerves are among the nervous system components that might be impacted by pathological alterations. Numerous clinical symptoms, including altered mental state, motor and sensory impairments, pain, or autonomic dysfunction, are frequently brought on by these changes. Impairment of blood supply to the brain causes conditions such as stroke, whereas gradual loss of neurons is the cause of neurodegenerative disorders like Parkinson's and Alzheimer's.

Understanding the mechanisms behind these neurological disorders is crucial for effective diagnosis, management, and the development of therapeutic strategies.

Basic Neuroanatomy and Function

The peripheral nervous system (PNS) and the central nervous system (CNS) comprise the nervous system. The brain and spinal cord, which are the main control centers for information processing and directing body activities, make up the central nervous system (CNS).

The cerebellum, brainstem, and cerebrum are the three main components of the brain. The most important component, the cerebrum, is in charge of higher order processes including memory, reasoning, emotion, voluntary movement, and sensory perception. While the brainstem controls vital autonomic processes like breathing, blood pressure, and heart rate, the cerebellum is in charge of balance and coordination.

Signals from the brain are sent to the body's other organs via the spinal cord, which serves as a communication highway. It regulates motor reactions and reflexes. The nerves that emerge from the brain and spinal cord and transmit information to and from the central nervous system (CNS) to other body areas make up the peripheral nervous system. It consists of the autonomic system, which manages involuntary processes like digestion and heartbeat, and the physiological system, which governs voluntary actions. Together, these elements sustain regular physiological reactions and processes.

Critical Conditions and Management:

Stroke, traumatic brain injury (TBI), and neurodegenerative disorders like Parkinson's and Alzheimer's are among the critical situations that can damage the nervous system. For each, a different care strategy is needed to alleviate symptoms and stop more harm.

When blood supply to a portion of the brain is cut off, cell death results, which is what happens in a stroke. Management focuses on rapid intervention. In the case of ischemic stroke, thrombolytic medications (clot busters) are administered to restore blood flow. Physical, occupational, and speech therapy rehabilitation is crucial for recovery and improving motor and cognitive functions.

Traumatic Brain Injury (TBI) is the outcome of brain injury brought on by an outside source. Stabilizing the patient, lowering intracranial pressure, and halting more damage are all part of management. Surgery can be required in extreme circumstances to remove clots or fix fractures. Improving cognitive function and physical capacities are the main goals of long-term rehabilitation.

Nerve cells gradually disappear in neurodegenerative illnesses like Parkinson's and Alzheimer's. For Parkinson's, management includes medications like levodopa to manage motor symptoms and physical therapy. Alzheimer's disease management focuses on symptom control with medications like cholinesterase inhibitors, cognitive therapies, and lifestyle modifications to support daily functioning.

Early diagnosis, tailored treatment, and ongoing management are vital in addressing these neurological conditions and enhancing patients' quality of life.

Stroke (Ischemic, Hemorrhagic):

A stroke is an abrupt interruption of blood flow to the brain that may cause damage to brain tissue. Hemorrhagic and ischemic are the two primary kinds.

Approximately 85% of all strokes are of the ischemic kind, which is the most prevalent kind. It happens when a blood clot obstructs a brain artery, stopping the blood flow. A thrombus, or clot that originates in the brain, or an embolus, or clot that moves from another region of the body, can cause this obstruction. The goal of management is to rapidly restore blood flow, and thrombolytic drugs such as tissue plasminogen activator (tPA) are frequently used if given within a certain amount of time. To physically remove the clot, mechanical thrombectomy may be used in some situations.

A burst blood artery in the brain causes hemorrhagic stroke, which is characterized by bleeding and elevated pressure on the brain's structures. This type of stroke can be caused by conditions like high blood pressure, aneurysms, or arteriovenous malformations (AVMs). Management aims to control the bleeding, reduce intracranial pressure, and stabilize the patient. Surgical interventions, such as clipping or coiling of an aneurysm, may be necessary.

To reduce brain damage, both forms of stroke require emergency medical intervention. Physical, occupational, and speech therapy are all parts of rehabilitation, which is essential for restoring lost capabilities and enhancing quality of life.

Pathophysiology: Atherosclerosis, Embolism, Hemorrhage

An important factor in ischemic stroke is atherosclerosis. The accumulation of fatty deposits in the artery walls causes atherosclerosis, which narrows the arteries and lowers blood flow to the brain. On these plaques, a blood clot (thrombus) has the potential to impede blood flow and cause a stroke. An embolism happens when debris or blood clot from elsewhere in the body— usually the heart—moves to the brain, obstructing a blood artery and resulting in an ischemic episode.

The pathophysiology of hemorrhagic stroke is the rupture of a weak blood artery, which is frequently brought on by arteriovenous malformations (AVMs), aneurysms, or excessive blood pressure. The bleeding that follows raises intracranial pressure, compresses brain tissue, and interferes with normal blood flow, all of which cause cell death.

Clinical Features

The part of the brain that is damaged determines the clinical characteristics of a stroke. Shared focal neurological deficits refer to impairments in certain neurological functions such as movement, feeling, or vision. If a stroke damages the language centers in the brain, it may result in aphasia, which impairs speaking and comprehension of speech. Another characteristic of a stroke is hemiplegia, or paralysis on one side of the body, which frequently denotes damage to the motor cortex. Acknowledging these characteristics is essential for a timely diagnosis and treatment to minimize long-term consequences.

Diagnostic Workup

Diagnostic workup for stroke involves a combination of imaging studies and clinical assessments to determine the stroke's type, location, and severity.

Usually, a CT scan is the initial imaging test carried out. It recognizes brain bleeding to promptly identify hemorrhagic strokes. Even though a CT scan may not reveal any abnormalities right away in an ischemic stroke, it is essential for ruling out bleeding before starting some therapies, such as thrombolysis.

An MRI provides a more detailed view of brain tissue and can detect ischemic stroke in its early stages. It is instrumental in identifying small or deep brain infarcts that may not be visible on a CT scan.

Healthcare professionals use the NIH Stroke Scale, a standardized instrument, to determine the severity of a stroke. It assesses a range of neurological abilities, including speech, motor skills, awareness, and feeling. The scale offers a starting point for monitoring patient development and aids in guiding treatment decisions.

Management

The main therapy for ischemic stroke is thrombolysis with tissue plasminogen activator (tPA) provided it is given within a certain window of time (usually between 3-4.5 hours after symptom onset). By dissolving the blood clot, thrombolysis minimizes brain damage and restores blood flow. Aspirin is one antiplatelet medication that stops new clot formation. In certain situations, a mechanical thrombectomy may be necessary to manually remove the clot from a significant artery.

The goals of hemorrhagic stroke treatment are to lower intracranial pressure and reduce bleeding. Medication, surgery, or techniques like coiling or cutting aneurysms may be used in this.

An essential component of managing a stroke is rehabilitation. It seeks to enhance patients' quality of life and assist them in regaining lost functions. It consists of speech, occupational, and physical treatment based on the requirements of the patient.

Traumatic Brain Injury (TBI):

When an external force, such as a knock to the head, impairs normal brain function, it results in traumatic brain injury (TBI). Falling, driving accidents, sports injuries, and assaults are common causes. TBI can cause deficits in behavior, cognition, and physical functioning, ranging from minor concussions to severe cases. Symptoms vary based on the injury's severity and may include headaches, confusion, memory loss, dizziness, or loss of consciousness. Management involves stabilizing the patient, reducing intracranial pressure, and preventing further injury. Surgery can be necessary in extreme circumstances to remove clots or release pressure. The goals of rehabilitation are to enhance quality of life and restore function.

Types

When an external force, such as a knock to the head, impairs normal brain function, it results in traumatic brain injury (TBI). Falling, driving accidents, sports injuries, and assaults are common causes. TBI can cause deficits in behavior, cognition, and physical functioning, ranging from minor concussions to severe cases. Symptoms vary based on the injury's severity and may include headaches, confusion, memory loss, dizziness, or loss of consciousness. Management involves stabilizing the patient, reducing intracranial pressure, and preventing further injury. Surgery can be necessary in extreme circumstances to remove clots or release pressure. The goals of rehabilitation are to enhance quality of life and restore function.

Pathophysiology

Traumatic Brain Injury (TBI) pathophysiology involves both primary mechanical injury and secondary processes such as swelling.

Mechanical injury occurs at the moment of impact, directly damaging brain tissue, blood vessels, and nerve fibers. This impact can cause bruising (contusions), tearing (shearing) of brain tissue, or bleeding (hematomas), disrupting normal brain function.

Secondary swelling develops shortly after the initial injury. Damaged cells release inflammatory mediators, leading to brain swelling (edema) and increased intracranial pressure. This swelling further compresses brain tissue, restricts blood flow, and exacerbates neuronal damage. Secondary swelling is often more damaging than the initial impact, making prompt medical intervention crucial to limit ongoing injury.

Clinical Features

Depending on the extent of the injury, altered awareness, forgetfulness, and headaches are frequent clinical signs of traumatic brain injury (TBI).

Altered consciousness ranges from brief confusion to complete loss of consciousness (coma). Mild TBI, such as a concussion, may cause temporary disorientation, while severe TBI can lead to prolonged unconsciousness or a coma.

Amnesia is often present, with patients experiencing memory loss of the events immediately before (retrograde amnesia) or after (anterograde amnesia) the injury. This memory gap can help assess the injury's impact and severity.

Headache is a frequent symptom due to the direct impact on brain tissue and the increased intracranial pressure from swelling. Persistent or worsening headaches are red flags, indicating possible complications like bleeding or increased pressure.

Management: ICP Monitoring, Surgical Intervention

Management of Traumatic Brain Injury (TBI) focuses on preventing further brain damage and stabilizing the patient's condition.

Intracranial Pressure (ICP) monitoring is crucial, especially in moderate to severe TBI cases. Elevated ICP can result from swelling or bleeding in the brain, compressing vital structures and reducing blood flow. Monitoring helps guide interventions to maintain safe pressure levels, often using medications like mannitol or hypertonic saline to minimize swelling and prevent further injury.

Surgical intervention may be necessary when there is significant brain swelling, bleeding (hematoma), or skull fractures. Procedures like decompressive craniectomy relieve pressure by removing a portion of the skull, while hematoma evacuation clears blood clots to restore normal brain function. These measures aim to minimize brain damage and improve long-term outcomes.

Neurodegenerative Diseases (Parkinson's, Alzheimer's):

Progressive neuronal loss is a hallmark of neurodegenerative illnesses including Parkinson's and Alzheimer's, which impair cognitive and motor abilities.

Parkinson's disease predominantly affects the brain area responsible for controlling movement, the substantia nigra, which contains dopamine-producing neurons. This loss results in symptoms like tremors, muscle rigidity, bradykinesia (slowed movement), and postural instability. As the disease progresses, patients may also experience non-motor symptoms, including sleep disturbances, depression, and cognitive decline. Management focuses on medications like levodopa to supplement dopamine and improve motor function alongside physical therapy.

The buildup of tau tangles and beta-amyloid plaques in the brain, which causes a gradual loss of neurons and synapses, is a hallmark of Alzheimer's disease. This causes behavioral changes, disorientation, memory loss, trouble speaking and solving problems, and difficulties with language. Management involves medications such as cholinesterase inhibitors to temporarily improve cognitive symptoms and lifestyle interventions to support daily functioning. Both conditions require comprehensive, long-term care strategies to manage symptoms and enhance quality of life.

Pathophysiology: Protein Aggregation, Neuronal Death

Protein aggregation and consequent neuronal death are involved in the pathogenesis of neurodegenerative illnesses including Parkinson's and Alzheimer's.

Alpha-synuclein abnormally accumulates in Parkinson's disease and causes Lewy bodies, which are clumps in the neurons, especially in the substantia nigra. The buildup impairs regular cell activity, which causes dopamine-producing neurons to die. Dopamine deficiency affects the brain's capacity to control movement and coordination, leading to classic motor symptoms such as stiffness and tremors.

Tau and beta-amyloid are two aberrant proteins that build up in the brain during Alzheimer's disease. Communication between neurons is hampered by beta-amyloid plaques. Inside neurons, tau proteins tangle to hinder nutrition delivery and cause cell death. Memory loss, cognitive decline, and behavioral abnormalities are the outcomes of this gradual loss of neurons, especially in the hippocampal and cerebral cortex.

These protein aggregates and neuronal damage are central to the progression of both conditions, leading to the gradual worsening of motor and cognitive functions. Understanding these mechanisms helps guide the development of targeted treatments and management strategies.

Clinical Features: Tremors, Cognitive Decline, Rigidity

Tremors, stiffness, and cognitive decline are some of the unique clinical hallmarks of neurodegenerative illnesses including Parkinson's and Alzheimer's.

Tremors are a hallmark of Parkinson's disease. They typically begin as a rhythmic shaking in one hand, often noticed when the hand is at rest. As the disease progresses, tremors may affect other body parts, including the legs, jaw, or face, making everyday activities increasingly challenging.

Cognitive decline is most prominent in Alzheimer's disease but can also occur in the later stages of Parkinson's. It starts with mild memory lapses and difficulty concentrating and eventually progresses to problems with language, decision-making, and performing familiar tasks. Behavioral changes and confusion become more pronounced as the disease advances.

Rigidity refers to muscle stiffness experienced in Parkinson's disease, which affects movement and causes discomfort. It often leads to a stooped posture and a shuffling gait, further contributing to mobility issues. The bradykinesia (slowed movement), tremors, and rigidity have a substantial negative effect on the patient's quality of life. Early diagnosis and individualized treatment of these neurodegenerative disorders are made easier by the recognition of these clinical characteristics.

Management

Treatment for neurological disorders including stroke and Parkinson's disease frequently consists of a mix of drugs and treatments designed to target different symptoms.

Parkinson's disease is mostly treated with dopaminergic drugs, such as levodopa. These drugs assist to reduce motor symptoms including stiffness, tremors, and bradykinesia (slowness of movement) by raising dopamine levels in the brain. Other medications that control symptoms and enhance motor performance include dopamine agonists and MAO-B inhibitors. Adjusting medication doses over time is essential, as Parkinson's is a progressive condition that evolves in its presentation.

Cognitive therapies are crucial in managing the cognitive impairments associated with Parkinson's disease and stroke. Cognitive rehabilitation aims to strengthen patients' memory, attention, and problem-solving skills through structured exercises and strategies. Speech and language therapy can help those with aphasia after a stroke regain communication abilities. These therapies work alongside medications to enhance overall quality of life, support daily functioning, and promote recovery or slowing of symptom progression.

Quick Clinical Assessment Checklist

A quick clinical assessment for neurological conditions requires thoroughly examining reflexes, cranial nerves, and motor function. This assessment helps identify areas of dysfunction within the nervous system and offers crucial insights into the nature and location of neurological disorders.

Neurological Exam involves evaluating several components:

Reflexes: Reflex testing is a vital part of the neurological Exam. Common reflexes tested include the patellar (knee-jerk), Achilles, biceps, and triceps reflexes. These tests involve tapping the tendons with a reflex hammer to observe the body's involuntary responses. Abnormal reflexes can indicate damage to specific areas of the nervous system. Exaggerated reflexes, or hyperreflexia, are indicative of upper motor neuron lesions, which are frequently observed in disorders such as multiple sclerosis and stroke. On the other hand, lack of reflexes or hyporeflexia indicate damage to the lower motor neurons, maybe as a result of spinal cord injury or peripheral neuropathy. Reflex testing offers a rapid summary of the peripheral and central nervous systems' integrity.

Cranial Nerves: All 12 cranial nerves are examined as part of a comprehensive neurological evaluation as they regulate sensation, movement, and autonomic processes in the head and neck. A brief assessment of the cranial nerves might consist of:

Cranial Nerve II (Optic): Testing visual acuity using a Snellen chart and checking visual fields can reveal issues such as optic neuropathy or intracranial pressure changes.

Cranial Nerves III, IV, and VI (Oculomotor, Trochlear, Abducens): Checking eye movements and pupil responses to light can detect abnormalities like ptosis (drooping eyelid), nystagmus (involuntary eye movements), or anisocoria (unequal pupil sizes), which may indicate brainstem pathology.

Cranial Nerve VII (Facial): Observing facial symmetry and expressions, such as smiling or frowning, helps identify facial nerve palsy, which may result from stroke or Bell's palsy.

Cranial Nerve IX and X (Glossopharyngeal and Vagus): Asking the patient to say "ah" while observing the movement of the uvula checks the integrity of these nerves. Abnormalities may suggest brainstem damage.

Quick cranial nerve testing provides immediate clues to brainstem or higher neural pathway involvement, assisting in localizing lesions.

Motor Function: Evaluating muscular strength, tone, and coordination in various body areas is part of the process of assessing motor function.

Strength: Asking the patient to push against resistance or perform simple movements like lifting their arms or legs tests muscle strength. Weakness (paresis) can indicate motor cortex, brainstem, spinal cord, or peripheral nerve lesions.

Tone: Passive movement of the limbs helps assess muscle tone. Increased tone, or spasticity, often points to upper motor neuron damage, as seen in stroke or multiple sclerosis. Conversely, reduced tone (flaccidity) may indicate lower motor neuron or peripheral nerve injury.

Coordination: Testing coordination through simple tasks, like touching the nose with an index finger or performing rapid alternating movements, assesses cerebellar function. Impaired coordination may suggest cerebellar ataxia or other neurological disorders.

By conducting a comprehensive neurological exam focused on reflexes, cranial nerves, and motor function, healthcare providers can rapidly identify neurological abnormalities, guiding further diagnostic testing and management. This quick yet detailed assessment is crucial in emergencies, such as stroke, where prompt recognition and intervention significantly impact outcomes.

CHAPTER 7: PEDIATRICS AND GERIATRICS

Pediatrics and geriatrics represent two distinct ends of the age spectrum, each with unique health considerations and challenges. In pediatrics, care focuses on growth, development, and the early detection of congenital or acute conditions, such as asthma and acute gastroenteritis. Children's bodies respond differently to illness and treatment, requiring careful attention to dosing, growth milestones, and immune system development. Geriatrics, on the other hand, involves managing chronic diseases, age-related changes, and the complexities of polypharmacy. Older adults often face conditions like dementia, osteoarthritis, and frailty, necessitating a comprehensive approach to maintain their quality of life and independence. Understanding the specific medical needs of both age groups is crucial for delivering age-appropriate care.

Pediatric Conditions:

Pediatric conditions often present unique characteristics and challenges requiring specialized care tailored to children's developing bodies and immune systems. Three common issues in pediatric care include asthma, acute gastroenteritis, and febrile seizures. A thorough pediatric assessment also involves tracking growth, monitoring vital signs, and evaluating developmental milestones to ensure children are progressing healthily.

Common Issues

One of the most common long-term illnesses in children is asthma. It causes inflammation and constriction of the airways, resulting in symptoms including tightness in the chest, coughing, wheezing, and shortness of breath. Pediatric asthma can be brought on by allergens, respiratory illnesses, exertion, and environmental factors. Severe exacerbations must be avoided by early detection and treatment. Treatment usually consists of long-term control drugs, such inhaled corticosteroids, to treat chronic inflammation and short-term bronchodilators, like albuterol, for acute symptoms. When it comes to recognizing triggers and giving recommended drugs, parents and other caregivers are essential in preserving the respiratory health of the kid.

Another frequent pediatric illness that is marked by intestinal and stomach irritation is acute gastroenteritis. Symptoms include nausea, vomiting, diarrhea, stomach discomfort, and occasionally fever.

Viral infections like rotavirus or norovirus often cause the condition, but bacteria and parasites can also be culprits. The primary concern in pediatric gastroenteritis is dehydration, as children can lose fluids rapidly. Treatment focuses on rehydration through oral rehydration solutions (ORS) containing balanced electrolytes and glucose. Intravenous fluids could be required in extreme situations. Preventive measures, including proper hand hygiene and rotavirus vaccination, are essential in reducing the incidence of acute gastroenteritis in children.

Fever in children, usually between the ages of six months and five years, is linked to febrile seizures. They are often frightening for parents but are generally harmless and do not indicate a severe neurological condition. Febrile seizures usually manifest as brief, generalized convulsions triggered by a rapid rise in body temperature, often during an infection. Management involves treating the underlying fever with antipyretics like acetaminophen and reassuring parents. While most febrile seizures do not require long-term treatment, repeated or complex seizures may warrant further evaluation by a healthcare professional.

Pediatric Assessment: Growth Charts, Vital Signs, Developmental Milestones

A comprehensive pediatric assessment is vital in identifying and managing these conditions. Growth charts monitor a child's growth pattern, comparing height, weight, and head circumference to standard percentiles for age and sex. Deviations from expected growth can signal underlying health issues, such as nutritional deficiencies or chronic illnesses.

Vital signs are another important way to assess a child's health. The normal ranges for blood pressure, heart rate, and respiratory rate in children vary according to age. For example, infants typically have faster heart rate and respiratory rate than older children. Regular monitoring helps detect early signs of illness or distress.

Developmental milestones provide insight into a child's physical, social, and cognitive development. Assessing milestones, such as sitting up, walking, speaking, and social interaction, helps identify delays that may suggest developmental disorders or neurological issues. Early detection through regular assessment enables timely intervention, improving long- term outcomes for children with developmental concerns.

Understanding common pediatric conditions and conducting thorough assessments allows healthcare providers to offer tailored, age-appropriate care that supports healthy growth and development.

Geriatric Conditions:

Geriatric conditions present unique challenges in healthcare due to the physiological changes associated with aging and the presence of multiple, often chronic, health conditions. In the aged population, polypharmacy, osteoarthritis, and dementia are among the most prevalent conditions. A comprehensive strategy that takes into account both the medical elements of these illnesses as well as the social, emotional, and functional requirements of older persons is needed to manage them.

Common Issues: Dementia, Osteoarthritis, Polypharmacy

A gradual neurological condition called dementia is typified by a loss of cognitive abilities including remembering, thinking, and speaking. It has a big influence on freedom and daily living. Alzheimer's disease is the most prevalent kind of dementia, with vascular dementia— which is frequently associated with stroke or other cardiovascular issues—coming in second. Early symptoms may include forgetfulness, difficulty finding words, and difficulty with complex tasks. As dementia worsens, people may become disoriented, exhibit personality changes, have poor judgment, and lose the capacity to carry out everyday tasks.

Dementia management involves several aspects. Memantine and other cholinesterase inhibitors, like as donepezil, can help temporarily control symptoms and moderate the rate of cognitive deterioration, even though there is no known treatment. Non-pharmacological interventions play a crucial role, including cognitive therapy, structured routines, and environmental modifications to enhance safety and comfort. Support for caregivers is equally essential, as dementia care can be demanding. In the later stages, planning for long-term care, such as in- home assistance or nursing facilities, becomes necessary. Addressing behavioral symptoms like agitation and aggression requires a sensitive approach, often involving behavioral strategies and environmental adjustments to reduce stressors.

Osteoarthritis is a degenerative joint condition that causes pain, stiffness, and limited movement in the joints due to the deterioration of cartilage. It can occur in any joint, although it usually affects weight-bearing joints including the spine, hips, and knees. Osteoarthritis is more common as people age, particularly in those who have a history of joint injury, obesity, or a family history of the condition. Joint discomfort that becomes worse with movement, stiffness following periods of inactivity, and edema surrounding the afflicted joints are some of the symptoms.

Pain relief, better joint function, and preservation of quality of life are the goals of osteoarthritis management. The cornerstone of treatment consists of non-pharmacological therapies, such as physical therapy to strengthen the muscles around the joints and frequent low-impact exercises like swimming and walking. Weight management is crucial in reducing joint stress, particularly for individuals with osteoarthritis of the knees or hips. Assistive devices like canes or walkers can also help alleviate pressure on affected joints, improving mobility.

Pain management typically involves the use of medications such acetaminophen and nonsteroidal anti-inflammatory medicines (NSAIDs). Localized pain can be relieved by topical therapies, such as capsaicin creams, with fewer adverse systemic effects. Intra-articular corticosteroid injections as a means of reducing pain and inflammation can be considered in more severe situations. For individuals who do not respond to conservative therapy, surgical procedures such joint replacement (e.g., knee or hip arthroplasty) can greatly improve function and reduce pain. However, surgery is typically reserved for those with advanced disease and significant functional impairment, and the decision must weigh the potential benefits against surgical risks, especially in older adults with multiple health issues.

The elderly frequently have many chronic diseases, which leads to daily polypharmacy—the concurrent use of multiple drugs. Although taking medicine is frequently required to treat illnesses including diabetes, arthritis, and hypertension, polypharmacy raises the risk of drug interactions, adverse drug events, and non-adherence to prescribed dosages. As the body's metabolism changes with age, older adults become more susceptible to the effects of medications, which can lead to complications such as falls, cognitive impairment, and hospitalizations.

Healthcare professionals must regularly examine patients' medications to determine the need, efficacy, and safety of each prescription in order to effectively manage polypharmacy. One of the most important aspects of providing care for the elderly is deprescribing, which is the act of tapering or stopping drugs that may no longer be necessary or that have more hazards than benefits. Providers need to take the patient's general health state, potential drug-drug interactions, and changes in kidney and liver function into account when modifying prescription regimens.

Non-pharmacological strategies are also emphasized to minimize medication reliance. For example, lifestyle modifications like diet and exercise can help manage conditions such as hypertension and diabetes, potentially reducing the need for multiple medications. Additionally, educating patients and caregivers about the proper use of drugs, including dosing schedules and potential side effects, can improve adherence and reduce the risk of adverse effects. Pharmacists' involvement in medication management adds an extra degree of security by making sure prescriptions are suitable and spotting possible conflicts.

In managing geriatric conditions, a holistic, patient-centered approach is crucial. For those with dementia, this involves supporting cognitive function, addressing behavioral symptoms, and providing caregiver support. Osteoarthritis includes combining physical therapy, lifestyle changes, pain management, and, when necessary, surgical intervention to maintain mobility and quality of life. Addressing polypharmacy requires careful medication review, deprescribing where possible, and emphasizing non-pharmacological interventions. Together, these strategies help improve outcomes and enhance the well-being of older adults, allowing them to maintain independence and a better quality of life.

Geriatric Assessment: Functional Status, Frailty Index, Cognitive Testing

A comprehensive geriatric assessment is essential for understanding the health status and needs of older adults. It goes beyond just addressing medical conditions. Key components include evaluating functional status, frailty, and cognitive function. This multifaceted approach aids in directing actions that are suited to the wellbeing of each individual and work to preserve their freedom and standard of living.

The capacity of a person to carry out instrumental activities of daily living (IADLs) and activities of daily living (ADLs) is the main emphasis of the functional status evaluation. While IADLs include more sophisticated activities like managing money, cooking, using the phone, and taking prescriptions, ADLs cover fundamental self-care chores like eating, dressing, bathing, and using the restroom. Assessing functional status helps identify the level of support a person might need, ranging from minimal assistance to full-time care. It provides insight into how conditions like osteoarthritis or dementia may impact daily life, guiding appropriate interventions such as physical therapy, assistive devices, or home care services.

The Frailty Index evaluates the susceptibility of older adults to unfavorable health consequences. Reduced strength, endurance, and physiological function are signs of frailty, which increases a person's risk of falling, being admitted to the hospital, and experiencing a general decline in health. A number of characteristics are taken into consideration while calculating the index, such as inadvertent weight loss, weakness, weariness, slowness, and poor physical activity. A higher score on the frailty index indicates an increased risk of complications and poorer health outcomes. Identifying frailty is crucial in tailoring care, as these individuals may require more careful monitoring, nutrition support, exercise programs to improve strength, and a cautious approach to medical interventions, such as surgery or medication changes.

Given the high frequency of cognitive decline and disorders like dementia in older persons, cognitive testing is an essential component of geriatric evaluation. The Mini-Mental State Examination (MMSE) and the Montreal Cognitive Assessment (MoCA) are common cognitive exams. These instruments assess memory, attention, language, executive function, and other components of cognitive function. Cognitive testing helps identify early signs of dementia or other cognitive impairments, allowing for timely interventions that can slow progression and support mental functioning. The assessment guides care planning for individuals experiencing cognitive decline, involving caregivers in medication management, providing memory aids, and creating a safe home environment.

Evaluating functional status, frailty, and cognitive function form a comprehensive picture of an older adult's health. Healthcare professionals may create tailored care plans that address medical and functional requirements, encourage independence, and enhance overall quality of life thanks to this comprehensive evaluation.

Quick Management Tips for Specific Populations

When managing health conditions in different age groups, especially in pediatrics and geriatrics, healthcare providers must consider age-specific factors that affect diagnosis, treatment, and overall care strategies. Each population has unique physiological characteristics, responses to medication, and psychosocial needs that influence how health conditions should be approached and managed effectively. Tailoring care to these considerations can significantly enhance patient outcomes, ensure safety, and improve the quality of life.

Pediatric Population

Children's bodies are constantly growing and developing, which presents unique challenges in medical treatment. Pediatric care requires a comprehensive understanding of how age, size, and developmental stage influence drug metabolism, disease presentation, and treatment response.

Medication Dosage and Administration

In pediatrics, dosing calculations are not standardized; they are based on a child's weight (in kilograms) and, in some cases, their body surface area. This weight-based dosing helps to avoid over- or under-medicating, which is crucial because children metabolize drugs differently than adults. For instance, infants and young children have a higher metabolic rate, which may require adjusted dosing schedules. Additionally, the liver and kidneys of children are not fully mature, affecting how medications are processed and excreted. Therefore, healthcare providers must exercise caution with drugs that have narrow therapeutic windows or are excreted primarily through the kidneys.

Liquid formulations or chewable tablets are often necessary for young children who may resist swallowing pills. Educating caregivers on how to measure and administer these forms correctly is equally important, as errors in dosing are more common with liquid medications.

Growth and Development Monitoring

Pediatrics treatment plans must also include regularly monitoring growth and developmental milestones. Chronic conditions, such as asthma or congenital heart disease, can impact a child's growth trajectory. Long-term use of medications like corticosteroids can affect growth rates, necessitating careful dose adjustments and monitoring. Providers must balance the benefits of managing the condition with potential side effects on the child's physical and cognitive development.

Vaccination and Preventive Care

Preventive care is a cornerstone of pediatric management. Immunization schedules should be followed diligently to protect children from infectious diseases, as their immune systems are still developing. In children with chronic conditions like asthma or diabetes, additional vaccinations, such as the annual influenza vaccine, are recommended to prevent complications. Education is essential, focusing on long-term health-promoting lifestyle practices including injury prevention, physical activity, and a balanced diet, for both the kid and the caregivers (when appropriate).

Geriatric Population

The senior population, comprising individuals aged 65 and older, presents different challenges. Aging affects the body's physiology, altering drug pharmacokinetics, increasing susceptibility to chronic diseases, and complicating clinical presentations. Management in this age group focuses on optimizing care while minimizing risks, such as polypharmacy and functional decline.

Medication Management and Polypharmacy

Elderly patients often manage multiple chronic conditions, leading to polypharmacy—the use of various medications concurrently. Due to age-related changes in medication metabolism, including diminished hepatic and renal function; older adults are more vulnerable to toxicity, interactions, and negative drug responses. Medications well-tolerated earlier in life may need dosage adjustments or even discontinuation to avoid complications.

A critical aspect of senior care is regular medication review, known as "deprescribing." This involves evaluating each drug's necessity, effectiveness, and safety in a patient's regimen. Non-essential medications, especially those with sedative effects or high fall risk, should be tapered off when possible. Healthcare providers should prioritize medicines that significantly impact quality of life and symptom control, using the "start low, go slow" approach for initiating or adjusting therapy.

Functional Status and Fall Prevention

Maintaining functional independence is a primary goal in senior care. Age-related changes, such as decreased muscle strength, balance issues, and joint stiffness, increase the risk of falls, leading to significant morbidity. Therefore, interventions to improve mobility, strength, and balance are crucial. These may include physical therapy, muscle-strengthening exercises, and assistive devices like walkers or canes.

Making changes to the surroundings at home might also lower the chance of falls. Simple but efficient solutions include removing trip hazards, adding grab bars to restrooms, and making sure there is enough illumination. Additionally, regular vision and hearing assessment can identify sensory impairments that may contribute to falls. Vitamin D supplementation may also be recommended to support bone health and reduce fall risk in elderly patients with osteoporosis or limited sun exposure.

Cognitive and Emotional Well-being

It is common for older adults to have cognitive decline, which can lead to dementia or moderate cognitive impairment and make care more difficult. Caregivers must be involved in maintaining medication adherence and appropriate self-care for persons with cognitive impairment. Simplifying medication regimens, using pill organizers, and setting up reminders can aid adherence.

Another important factor is mental health, as older people are more likely to experience social isolation and sadness. Regular screening for depression and anxiety should be part of the management plan, and access to social support or therapy services can significantly improve emotional well-being. Incorporating activities that stimulate cognitive function, such as puzzles, reading, or social engagement, can help slow mental decline and improve quality of life.

Shared Considerations for Both Age Groups

Despite their differences, pediatric and geriatric populations share some considerations in their treatment approaches. For both groups, individualized care is essential. Treatment plans must consider each person's unique physiology, lifestyle, and psychosocial context. Involving family members or caregivers in decision-making is crucial to understanding, adherence, and support.

Furthermore, regular follow-up is vital in monitoring progress and adjusting treatments. Children require ongoing assessment of growth and development. At the same time, the elderly need continuous evaluation of functional status, cognitive health, and medication safety. Education tailored to each group's needs and comprehension levels helps promote self-care and prevent complications.

Managing pediatric and geriatric populations requires a tailored approach considering age- specific physiological, cognitive, and functional factors. Healthcare professionals may improve treatment outcomes and these vulnerable groups' quality of life by carefully evaluating patients, managing their medications, and emphasizing lifestyle and support networks from an integrated perspective.

CHAPTER 8: REPRODUCTIVE HEALTH

The physical, mental, and social aspects of the reproductive system are all included in reproductive health, which is an essential component of overall wellbeing. It includes the opportunity to have a fulfilling and safe sexual life, the freedom to make reproductive decisions, access to quality healthcare, and the appropriate functioning and health of the reproductive organs. In both males and females, reproductive health spans various stages of life, including puberty, reproductive years, and beyond. Common disorders that can have a major influence on mental health and quality of life include endometriosis, prostatitis, infertility, polycystic ovarian syndrome (PCOS), erectile dysfunction, and hormonal imbalances. In order to promote long-term reproductive wellbeing, it is vital to comprehend these diseases, their consequences, and the significance of early detection and treatment.

Critical Conditions in Reproductive Health:

Since reproductive health has an impact on one's physical, emotional, and social well-being, it is essential to one's total wellbeing. Various conditions can disrupt reproductive health, impacting fertility, hormonal balance, and sexual function. Some of the most common reproductive health conditions include polycystic ovary syndrome (PCOS), endometriosis, and infertility in females, and erectile dysfunction and prostatitis in males. Comprehending these ailments is essential for efficient diagnosis, treatment, and overall well-being.

Female

Reproductive

Health

Conditions

Polycystic Ovary

Syndrome

(PCOS)

One of the most common endocrine conditions affecting women who are fertile is PCOS. Hormonal imbalance, irregular menstrual periods, and numerous ovarian cysts are its defining features. Although the precise origin of PCOS is yet unknown, a mix of environmental and genetic variables, including as inflammation, increased androgens, and insulin resistance, are thought to be involved.

Numerous symptoms, including irregular or nonexistent periods, hirsutism (excessive hair growth), acne, weight gain, and thinning hair, are frequently experienced by women with PCOS. One of the main characteristics of PCOS is insulin resistance, which raises the risk of type

2 diabetes and metabolic syndrome. Additionally, the hormonal imbalance associated with PCOS can disrupt ovulation, making it a leading cause of infertility.

Management of PCOS focuses on addressing the individual symptoms and underlying metabolic issues. Menstrual cycle regulation and improved insulin sensitivity can be achieved by lifestyle changes including eating a balanced diet and getting frequent exercise. Hormonal contraceptives are among the medications that can help control menstrual cycles and lessen symptoms like hirsutism and acne. Letrozole or clomiphene citrate are examples of ovulation- inducing drugs that can be taken by individuals who are trying to get pregnant. Metformin is frequently recommended in situations where insulin resistance is severe in order to enhance insulin sensitivity and aid in weight management.

Endometriosis

Endometriosis is a chronic illness characterized by the growth of tissue on the ovaries, fallopian tubes, and pelvic lining that resembles the endometrium and develops outside the uterine cavity. Pain, inflammation, and the production of adhesions—scar tissue—are caused by this aberrant growth. Symptoms of endometriosis often include pelvic discomfort, unpleasant periods (dysmenorrhea), pain during sex, and heavy menstrual flow. In rare instances, the disturbance of normal pelvic anatomy may potentially be a contributing factor to infertility.

Though the precise etiology of endometriosis is unknown, possibilities include immune system failure, genetic susceptibility, and retrograde menstruation—a condition in which menstrual blood travels backward into the pelvic cavity. Clinical assessment, imaging methods such as ultrasonography, and occasionally surgery to directly see endometrial abnormalities are typically necessary for diagnosis.

Management of endometriosis aims to alleviate pain, manage symptoms, and address fertility concerns. Hormonal therapy (such as oral contraceptives, progestins, and GnRH agonists) can be used to reduce or stop menstruation and inhibit the development of endometrial tissue. Nonsteroidal anti-inflammatory medicines (NSAIDs) can be used to relieve discomfort. In extreme situations, endometrial lesions and adhesions may need to be surgically removed, which might increase fertility and lessen discomfort.

Infertility

The failure to conceive following a year of consistent, unprotected sexual activity is known as infertility. It affects both males and females and can result from various factors, including hormonal imbalances, ovulatory disorders, structural abnormalities (e.g., blocked fallopian tubes), age-related factors, and underlying health conditions like PCOS and endometriosis.

In females, common causes of infertility include ovulation disorders (such as PCOS), fallopian tube damage or blockage, endometriosis, and age-related decline in egg quality. Assisted reproductive technologies (ART) including in vitro fertilization (IVF), drugs to promote ovulation, lifestyle changes, or surgical procedures to address anatomical problems may all be part of the management, depending on the underlying reason.

Male Reproductive Health Conditions
ED, or erectile dysfunction

The inability to obtain or sustain an erection strong enough for fulfilling sexual performance is known as erectile dysfunction. It is a prevalent ailment, especially in males over 40, and may be brought on by lifestyle, psychological, or medical reasons. Cardiovascular illness, diabetes, hormone imbalances, nerve injury, and certain drugs are examples of physical reasons. Relationship problems, stress, anxiety, sadness, and other psychological variables can potentially exacerbate ED.

Finding and treating the underlying cause is a crucial part of ED management. A good diet, regular exercise, giving up smoking, and consuming less alcohol are all examples of lifestyle modifications that can greatly enhance erectile performance. Oral drugs that improve blood flow to the penis, such as phosphodiesterase-5 (PDE5) inhibitors (sildenafil, tadalafil), are frequently administered. If the illness is significantly influenced by stress, anxiety, or interpersonal issues, psychological counseling or treatment may be advised. Other therapies, like as surgery, penile injections, or vacuum erection devices, can be required in some situations.

Prostatitis

Prostatitis, a frequent urological illness in males, is defined as inflammation of the prostate gland. Acute bacterial prostatitis, chronic bacterial prostatitis, chronic pelvic pain syndrome (CPPS), and silent inflammatory prostatitis are the four categories into which it can be divided. Depending on the kind, symptoms can vary, but they frequently include fever and chills in acute instances, frequent urine, painful urination, and pelvic discomfort.

The causes of prostatitis can range from bacterial infections to non-infectious factors such as muscle tension, nerve damage, or autoimmune responses. A physical examination, which includes a digital rectal exam (DRE), urine tests, and occasionally imaging scans to assess the prostate, are all part of the diagnosis process.

Management of prostatitis depends on the specific type. Acute bacterial prostatitis typically requires antibiotic therapy to clear the infection, while chronic bacterial prostatitis may need longer antibiotics. Treatment focuses on symptom relief for non-bacterial forms through medications like alpha-blockers (to relax prostate muscles), anti-inflammatory drugs, and lifestyle modifications. Physical therapy, stress reduction, and dietary changes can also help alleviate symptoms, particularly in chronic pelvic pain syndrome.

Conditions like PCOS, endometriosis, infertility, erectile dysfunction, and prostatitis present unique challenges in reproductive health. To ensure better quality of life and reproductive results, effective care necessitates a comprehensive strategy that treats both physical symptoms and underlying reasons. For both males and females, controlling symptoms, promoting fertility, and improving general reproductive health depend heavily on early diagnosis and intervention.

Clinical Assessment:

For the purpose of detecting and treating disorders that impact both men and women, a comprehensive clinical evaluation of reproductive health is essential. This procedure include gathering a thorough medical history from the patient and conducting a targeted physical examination. Knowing the important historical questions to ask and the physical exam areas to check can help medical professionals diagnose patients more accurately and provide individualized treatment plans.

Key History Questions

In order to evaluate the state of reproductive health, a thorough history must be obtained. Depending on the patient's gender and individual symptoms or concerns, the questions change somewhat.

For Female Patients

When evaluating female patients, start by asking about menstrual history. Important questions include:

- The age at menarche (onset of periods).
- The regularity and duration of menstrual cycles.
- The volume of menstrual flow.
- The presence of symptoms such as severe cramping (dysmenorrhea) or irregular periods.

These details can provide valuable insights into conditions like polycystic ovary syndrome (PCOS) or endometriosis.

Sexual history is another crucial aspect, where patients should be asked about sexual activity, use of contraception, history of sexually transmitted infections (STIs), and any pain during intercourse (dyspareunia). These questions help identify possible infections, hormonal imbalances, or conditions affecting reproductive organs, such as pelvic inflammatory disease (PID) or endometriosis.

For patients presenting with fertility concerns, inquire about the duration of attempts to conceive, previous pregnancies, history of miscarriages, and any treatments or interventions previously attempted. Information on lifestyle factors, such as smoking, alcohol use, exercise habits, and weight changes, is also crucial, as these can impact reproductive health and fertility.

For Male Patients

In male patients, key history questions focus on sexual health and function. Questions about libido (sexual desire), erectile function, ejaculation problems, and any pain associated with sexual activity provide insight into issues such as erectile dysfunction (ED) or other sexual health disorders. It's also essential to ask about urinary symptoms like difficulty urinating, weak stream, urgency, or pain, which may indicate conditions like prostatitis.

Fertility history is another critical area. Questions about previous fertility testing, history of STIs, testicular injuries, or surgeries can point to possible causes of infertility. A thorough history of lifestyle choices, such as drinking alcohol, smoking, using drugs, and being exposed to work-related risks, can also be used to pinpoint outside influences on reproductive health.

For both male and female patients, discussing family history of reproductive health issues, hormonal disorders, cancers (such as breast, ovarian, or prostate cancer), and genetic conditions is essential, as these can influence risk assessments and management plans.

Physical Exam Points

A targeted physical examination—which differs depending on the patient's sex and presenting symptoms—follows the history to reveal further information about the patient's reproductive health status.

For Female Patients

A female physical exam often begins with a general inspection, noting signs such as abnormal hair growth (hirsutism), acne, or obesity, which may suggest hormonal imbalances like those seen in PCOS. Given the thyroid's impact on menstrual cycles and fertility, a thyroid exam may be included to assess for thyroid enlargement or nodules.

A pelvic examination is crucial for evaluating reproductive organs. It includes an external inspection for signs of lesions, discharge, or abnormalities. During the internal exam, the healthcare provider assesses the vagina, cervix, uterus, and adnexa (ovaries and fallopian tubes). Palpation helps detect abnormalities like uterine fibroids, ovarian cysts, or tenderness indicative of infections or endometriosis. A Pap smear may be performed to screen for cervical cancer, and swabs can be taken to test for STIs.

For Male Patients

In males, the physical exam involves both a general assessment and a focused genital examination. A general inspection includes checking for signs such as gynecomastia (enlarged breast tissue) or body habitus changes that may indicate hormonal imbalances. The abdomen and flank regions are examined to identify any masses or tenderness.

The genital examination involves inspection and palpation of the penis, scrotum, testicles, and prostate. The provider looks for signs such as penile lesions, urethral discharge, and testicular abnormalities (e.g., masses, varicoceles). Testicular size, consistency, and tenderness are evaluated, as changes can suggest conditions like testicular cancer, hydrocele, or varicocele, which may impact fertility. A digital rectal exam (DRE) assesses the prostate gland. The provider checks for prostate size, tenderness, nodules, or irregularities during the DRE. When assessing symptoms associated with prostate cancer, benign prostatic hyperplasia (BPH), or prostatitis, this is very crucial.

Additional Assessments

Regardless of the patient's sex, additional assessments may include measuring vital signs, especially blood pressure, as part of a cardiovascular health check, given the interplay between cardiovascular and reproductive health (e.g., erectile dysfunction can be linked to heart disease). Since obesity is a risk factor for several reproductive disorders, such as PCOS, infertility, and erectile dysfunction, weight and BMI are also examined.

In reproductive health assessments, gathering detailed information through history-taking and performing a focused physical exam is essential to understanding the underlying conditions. For females, the emphasis is on menstrual history, sexual health, and a thorough pelvic exam, while for males, sexual function, urinary symptoms, and genital and prostate evaluations are essential. This holistic approach guides healthcare providers in making accurate diagnoses and developing individualized treatment plans, ensuring that reproductive health's physical and emotional aspects are addressed effectively.

Management Essentials

Managing disorders related to reproductive health necessitates an all-encompassing strategy that involves lifestyle changes, hormone therapies, and even surgical procedures. Each option addresses specific aspects of reproductive health, aiming to alleviate symptoms, restore normal functioning, and improve overall quality of life.

Hormonal Treatments

Hormonal treatments are often the first line of therapy for many reproductive conditions, particularly those resulting from hormonal imbalances.

Hormonal therapies are commonly employed for female patients to address problems such as endometriosis, irregular menstruation, and polycystic ovarian syndrome (PCOS). Oral contraceptives with progestin and estrogen are frequently used for PCOS in order to control menstrual cycles, lower testosterone levels, and treat symptoms including acne and hirsutism (excessive hair growth). Furthermore, normal menstrual flow can be induced with progestin medication alone, which lowers the risk of endometrial hyperplasia. Hormonal therapies, including progestins, gonadotropin-releasing hormone (GnRH) agonists, and oral contraceptives, can help women with endometriosis manage their pain and inflammation by slowing the development of endometrial tissue and suppressing the menstrual cycle.

Medication like letrozole or clomiphene citrate is used to stimulate ovulation in situations of infertility brought on by hormonal problems such ovulatory dysfunction. Furthermore, in more complicated situations, injectable gonadotropins may be used, frequently in combination with assisted reproductive technologies (ART) such as in vitro fertilization (IVF).

For males, hormonal treatments are also essential in managing specific conditions. Erectile dysfunction (ED) can sometimes be related to low testosterone levels. In such cases, testosterone replacement therapy (TRT) may help restore sexual function and improve libido. However, TRT must be carefully monitored due to potential side effects, including the risk of exacerbating prostate conditions.

Lifestyle Modifications

Making lifestyle adjustments is essential for addressing diseases related to reproductive health, particularly when underlying problems like stress, nutrition, and weight are involved.

Changes in lifestyle can greatly reduce symptoms and enhance general health for women who suffer from illnesses like PCOS or endometriosis. Weight management, improved insulin sensitivity, and hormone regulation may all be achieved with a balanced diet full of fruits, vegetables, whole grains, and lean meats, as well as regular physical exercise. For women with PCOS, weight loss—even as little as 5–10% of total body weight—can improve ovulation and menstrual regularity, which increases the likelihood of pregnancy. Stress can worsen the symptoms of illnesses related to reproductive health, thus practicing stress management practices like mindfulness, yoga, or counseling is also useful.

Changes in lifestyle are frequently necessary for both couples in the management of infertility. It is advised to follow a nutritious diet, keep a healthy weight, stop smoking, drink less alcohol, and manage stress. These adjustments enhance reproductive health and enhance the results of fertility therapies.

For males, lifestyle modifications are essential in addressing issues like erectile dysfunction and infertility. Healthy eating, getting enough sleep, and exercising on a regular basis can enhance blood flow and general health, which can enhance sexual performance. Smoking cessation is essential, as smoking can impair blood vessels and reduce sperm quality. Limiting alcohol consumption and avoiding substance abuse are also crucial in optimizing reproductive health. Men are advised to keep a healthy weight since obesity can cause hormone imbalances that impair fertility and sexual performance.

Surgical Options

Surgical interventions are considered when conservative treatments like hormonal therapy and lifestyle modifications are insufficient in managing symptoms or improving reproductive health.

In some cases of infertility and disorders such as endometriosis, female patients may require surgery. By removing or eliminating endometrial implants, cysts, and adhesions, laparoscopy is a minimally invasive surgical technique that is frequently used to diagnose and treat endometriosis. This surgery also improves fertility and relieves discomfort. In women with structural abnormalities, such as fibroids, polyps, or blocked fallopian tubes, surgical correction may enhance fertility. For example, a myomectomy is a procedure that removes uterine fibroids while preserving the uterus, which can be beneficial for women wishing to conceive.

In infertility cases related to fallopian tube blockage or scarring, surgical procedures like tubal reconstruction or adhesiolysis can help restore tubal patency, increasing the chances of natural conception. Additionally, surgical interventions such as ovarian drilling may be used in PCOS to stimulate ovulation when other treatments have failed.

For males, surgery is an option in cases of reproductive health issues like varicocele and certain forms of erectile dysfunction. A varicocelectomy involves the surgical removal or correction of a varicocele (enlarged veins within the scrotum), which can improve sperm quality and enhance fertility outcomes. In cases of erectile dysfunction related to penile blood flow, vascular surgery might be performed to improve blood circulation to the penis. Penile implants or prosthetic devices are also options for men with severe erectile dysfunction who are unresponsive to medication.

Surgery may also be necessary if prostatitis is not improved with antibiotics or other therapies. For instance, in patients with considerable prostate enlargement and persistent prostatitis, transurethral resection of the prostate (TURP) can help reduce symptoms related to urination.

Integrating Management Approaches

An integrated approach combining hormonal treatments, lifestyle modifications, and, if necessary, surgical interventions often yields the best outcomes in managing reproductive health conditions. Patients should be involved in decision-making, understanding the benefits and risks of each option. For example, women with PCOS may benefit from a combination of hormonal therapy, weight management, and possibly laparoscopic surgery to improve fertility. Similarly, men experiencing erectile dysfunction might see improvements through a mix of lifestyle changes, medications, and, if needed, surgical solutions.

Ultimately, the goal of these management strategies is to address symptoms, improve reproductive function, and enhance overall quality of life, tailored to each patient's individual needs. Regular follow-up and ongoing assessment are essential to adapting treatment plans as conditions evolve or improve.

CHAPTER 9: MATERNITY AND NEONATOLOGY

Maternity and neonatology focus on the health and well-being of the mother and the newborn, encompassing the period before, during, and after childbirth. Maternity care involves:

- Monitoring the physical and emotional health of the mother.
- Managing pregnancy-related conditions.
- Ensuring a safe delivery process.

This phase is crucial as it sets the foundation for the baby's health and development. Neonatology, on the other hand, deals with the medical care of newborns, particularly those who are premature, have low birth weight, or face different health challenges immediately after birth. Providing comprehensive care during these stages is vital to address complications, promote healthy growth, and support families in their transition to parenthood. Understanding the common conditions and management practices in maternity and neonatal care is essential for ensuring the best outcomes for mothers and their babies.

Maternity Care:

In order to protect both the mother's and the growing baby's health, maternity care entails the thorough treatment of a mother's health before to, during, and following pregnancy. Monitoring and treating illnesses that might develop during pregnancy, such as gestational diabetes and hypertensive disorders, is one of the most important parts of maternity care. Both conditions, if left unmanaged, can have significant implications for maternal and fetal health, highlighting the need for vigilant prenatal care and appropriate interventions.

Hypertensive Disorders of Pregnancy

Preeclampsia, chronic hypertension, gestational hypertension, and other illnesses fall under the category of hypertensive disorders, which are among the most prevalent pregnancy problems. If these problems are not detected and treated right once, the mother and child may be seriously at danger.

In women with previously normal blood pressure, gestational hypertension sets in after 20 weeks of pregnancy. When there is no proteinuria (protein in the urine), it is defined by a systolic blood pressure of 140 mm Hg or higher or a diastolic blood pressure of 90 mm Hg or higher.

While gestational hypertension often resolves after delivery, it requires close monitoring to prevent progression to preeclampsia or other complications such as preterm birth.

Preeclampsia, a more severe form of hypertensive illness, is characterized by elevated blood pressure and proteinuria. It usually appears after 20 weeks of pregnancy. Additional symptoms that may manifest include intense headaches, blurred vision, and hand and facial edema. Preeclampsia can affect multiple organ systems, leading to complications like liver dysfunction, kidney injury, and reduced blood flow to the placenta, which can impact fetal growth and development. Preeclampsia can progress to eclampsia, which is marked by convulsions, if treatment is not received. This might be fatal for the mother and the unborn child.

In order to avoid difficulties, careful prenatal monitoring and blood pressure control are the mainstays of management of hypertensive diseases in pregnancy. Along with routine monitoring, lifestyle changes including a balanced diet and moderate exercise are generally advised for mild gestational hypertension. In cases of preeclampsia, closer surveillance is necessary, which may include frequent blood pressure checks, urine tests, and fetal monitoring. Medications like antihypertensives (e.g., labetalol or methyldopa) may be prescribed to manage blood pressure, and corticosteroids are sometimes given to enhance fetal lung development if early delivery becomes necessary. Regardless of gestational age, delivery of the infant may be the only effective treatment in extreme circumstances to stop more difficulties for both the mother and the fetus.

Gestational Diabetes

Another prevalent pregnancy complication is gestational diabetes mellitus (GDM), which is defined by the development or discovery of glucose intolerance during pregnancy. Blood sugar levels rise as a result of the body's inability to create enough insulin to fulfill the needs of pregnancy. If left untreated, gestational diabetes can harm both the mother and the unborn child and usually appears in the second or third trimester.

Risk factors for gestational diabetes include:

- Obesity.
- Advanced maternal age.
- Family history of diabetes.
- A history of GDM in previous pregnancies.

Pregnant women who have gestational diabetes are more likely to get preeclampsia, high blood pressure, and cesarean birth. Uncontrolled blood sugar levels can cause macrosomia, or excessive fetal development, in the unborn child, which increases the chance of birth traumas and necessitates delivery measures. Furthermore, hypoglycemia, or low blood sugar, is a condition that newborns of moms with GDM are more likely to experience soon after birth. Later in age, they could be more likely to develop type 2 diabetes and obesity.

The focus of their gestational diabetes management is on preserving ideal blood glucose levels during pregnancy. The main tactics are lifestyle changes, such as eating a healthy diet, getting frequent exercise, and keeping an eye on blood sugar levels. In order to assist control blood sugar levels, women are frequently recommended to eat a diet high in fiber and low in simple carbohydrates. Insulin treatment or oral drugs like metformin may be administered to effectively control the illness if lifestyle adjustments alone are insufficient to keep blood glucose within the therapeutic range.

Regular prenatal visits are essential for monitoring both the mother and the baby. Healthcare providers often perform additional ultrasounds to assess fetal growth and amniotic fluid levels and tests to evaluate the baby's well-being, such as non-stress tests or biophysical profiles. Postpartum follow-up is also crucial, as women with gestational diabetes have an increased risk of developing type 2 diabetes later in life. Lifestyle interventions after pregnancy can help mitigate this risk, emphasizing the importance of long-term health maintenance.

Hypertensive disorders and gestational diabetes are significant conditions that require careful management during pregnancy. Early detection through prenatal screening, lifestyle modifications, medication when necessary, and close monitoring are crucial to minimizing risks and promoting healthy outcomes for both the mother and baby. Proper maternity care, involving regular prenatal visits and comprehensive assessments, ensures these conditions are managed effectively to support a safe pregnancy and delivery.

Neonatal Care:

The goal of neonatal care is to promote the health and wellbeing of infants, with a special emphasis on the crucial first 28 days of life, when major physiological changes occur. Some newborns, especially those born prematurely or with specific health issues, may face complications that require specialized care. Among the common conditions that can affect newborns are neonatal jaundice and respiratory distress syndrome (RDS). Proper identification and management of these conditions are crucial to ensuring the best possible outcomes for the infant.

Neonatal Jaundice

A common ailment in infants, neonatal jaundice is characterized by a yellow coloring of the skin and eyes. It is caused by an overabundance of the yellow pigment bilirubin, which is created naturally when red blood cells break down. The liver, which breaks down and excretes bilirubin, may not be completely developed in infants, which can cause a brief accumulation of bilirubin in the body.

Jaundice typically appears within the first few days of life and is usually harmless (physiological jaundice). However, in some cases, it may indicate more severe conditions, such as blood type incompatibility (Rh or ABO incompatibility), infections, or metabolic disorders. If bilirubin levels become excessively high, there is a risk of developing kernicterus, a form of brain damage that can lead to lifelong neurological issues.

The diagnosis of neonatal jaundice is primarily clinical, with healthcare providers assessing the newborn's skin and eye color. To quantify bilirubin levels and assess the degree of jaundice, a blood test is frequently used. The infant's age and bilirubin level determine how the condition is managed. In moderate instances, more frequent feedings are advised to enhance stooling and hydration, both of which aid in bilirubin elimination. For moderate to severe cases, phototherapy is the mainstay of treatment. In order to do this, the infant must be exposed to a certain kind of light, which changes bilirubin into a form that is easier to expel through urine and stool. An exchange transfusion may be required in rare circumstances where bilirubin levels are dangerously high and do not react to phototherapy in order to rapidly lower bilirubin levels.

Monitoring bilirubin levels and the infant's general well-being is crucial, as prompt treatment of neonatal jaundice can prevent complications and support healthy development. Follow-up visits after discharge are often recommended to ensure that bilirubin levels decrease and that the newborn continues to thrive.

Respiratory Distress Syndrome (RDS)

Premature babies are the main victims of respiratory distress syndrome (RDS), especially those born before 37 weeks of gestation. It is caused by the lungs' underdevelopment as well as a surfactant deficit, which lowers the lungs' surface tension and keeps the alveoli (air sacs) open. The alveoli collapse in the absence of sufficient surfactant, making it difficult for the baby to breathe and efficiently exchange oxygen.

Early respiratory distress symptoms in infants with RDS usually include grunting, flaring of the nostrils, rapid, shallow breathing (tachypnea), chest retractions (where the chest muscles visibly pull inward during breathing), and cyanosis (bluish discoloration of the skin due to low oxygen levels). Because younger babies' lungs are still developing, they are more susceptible to RDS, which is commonly correlated with the infant's gestational age.

A chest X-ray can corroborate the diagnosis of RDS, which is based on clinical presentation and often displays the lungs with a distinctive "ground-glass" look. Blood tests also monitor oxygen and carbon dioxide levels, ensuring the infant receives sufficient respiratory support.

RDS management calls for prompt medical attention from specialists. To keep the blood's oxygen levels at a healthy level, more oxygen is frequently given. Infants may require continuous positive airway pressure (CPAP), a non-invasive breathing technique that helps maintain open airways, in more severe situations. For newborns experiencing severe respiratory distress, mechanical ventilation may be required to assist breathing. One of the mainstays of RDS treatment is exogenous surfactant therapy, which involves breathing a synthetic or natural surfactant directly into the baby's lungs via a breathing tube. By stabilizing the alveoli, this therapy enhances gas exchange and breathing.

Preventive measures can also reduce the risk of RDS. For mothers at risk of preterm delivery, administering antenatal corticosteroids (such as betamethasone) can accelerate lung maturity in the fetus, increasing surfactant production and reducing the severity of RDS if preterm birth occurs.

Babies with RDS require constant observation since the disorder can cause long-term breathing problems or consequences including bronchopulmonary dysplasia (BPD). The prognosis for newborns with RDS has greatly improved with breakthroughs in neonatal care, and many have recovered completely with the right therapies.

Neonatal jaundice and respiratory distress syndrome are common conditions that require prompt and effective management to ensure healthy outcomes for newborns. Early identification, careful monitoring, and appropriate interventions, whether through phototherapy for jaundice or respiratory support and surfactant therapy for RDS, are vital to supporting the health and development of these vulnerable infants.

Quick Tips for Obstetric and Neonatal Emergencies

Managing obstetric and neonatal emergencies requires quick thinking and effective action to protect both mother and baby. Recognizing the warning signs early in cases of preeclampsia and eclampsia is essential. Symptoms like severe headaches, blurred vision or seeing spots, swelling in the hands and face, and high blood pressure often signal preeclampsia. If a pregnant woman shows signs of high blood pressure, typically measured at levels greater than 140/90 mm Hg, immediate action is required. Proteinuria, or protein in the urine, is also a critical indicator that needs to be checked regularly. Eclampsia, which is a more severe progression of preeclampsia, involves seizures and requires urgent treatment.

When managing preeclampsia, it is best to put the patient in a serene, stress-free setting to lower their chance of seizures. To regulate blood pressure, provide antihypertensive drugs such as hydralazine or labetalol. Magnesium sulfate is the recommended therapy for seizures in order to stop subsequent episodes, and emergency supplies should always be on hand in case things go out of control. Delivery may be necessary to protect both mother and baby, especially in severe cases. When preparing for delivery, an emergency cesarean section may be required, depending on the condition's progression.

In cases of postpartum hemorrhage, rapid intervention is essential. The signs of hemorrhage, such as excessive vaginal bleeding following childbirth, are an immediate red flag. First, check for uterine atony, which is when the uterus fails to contract effectively after delivery, a common cause of bleeding. Massage the uterus to encourage contractions and administer uterotonic agents like oxytocin to help control bleeding. If the bleeding persists, further interventions may include medications such as misoprostol or ergometrine to enhance uterine contractions.

Surgical intervention might be required if bleeding cannot be controlled through drugs and manual techniques. Swift action to manage blood loss, including fluid resuscitation or blood transfusion if necessary, is crucial in stabilizing the patient.

Another obstetric emergency is shoulder dystocia, where the baby's shoulder becomes stuck after the head has been delivered, obstructing the birth. The mother's pelvis can be widened and the impediment can be removed by performing the McRoberts procedure, which involves extending her legs firmly against her abdomen. Alternatively, suprapubic pressure may push the baby's shoulder downward and dislodge it. It's essential to remain calm and apply these techniques systematically while ensuring close communication with the medical team to facilitate a safe delivery.

In neonatal emergencies, recognizing and addressing respiratory distress is a priority, especially in preterm infants. If a newborn presents with rapid breathing, chest retractions, grunting, or cyanosis, immediate respiratory support is necessary. Administering oxygen or initiating continuous positive airway pressure (CPAP) helps maintain adequate oxygenation. In more severe cases, mechanical ventilation may be required. For infants with respiratory distress syndrome due to surfactant deficiency, administering surfactant therapy directly into the lungs can improve breathing and stabilize the infant's condition. Close monitoring of oxygen levels, respiratory rate, and overall stability is critical during these interventions.

Neonatal sepsis, another critical condition, presents with symptoms like lethargy, poor feeding, temperature instability, and rapid breathing. Early identification and immediate treatment are essential. Once sepsis is suspected, initiate broad-spectrum antibiotics immediately to cover the most likely pathogens. Blood cultures and other diagnostic tests should be taken to confirm the infection, but treatment should not be delayed while waiting for results. Close observation of the newborn's vital signs and supporting their hydration and oxygenation levels are essential in effectively managing sepsis.

In cases of neonatal resuscitation, it's vital to follow established guidelines. If a newborn is not breathing or has a weak heart rate after birth, initiate resuscitation with ventilation support, using a bag and mask to assist breathing. Chest compressions may be necessary if the heart rate remains low despite adequate ventilation. Adrenaline administration can be considered if the infant's condition does not improve with essential resuscitation efforts. Ensure that the newborn's airway remains open and provide thermal support to prevent hypothermia. Executed rapidly and efficiently, these steps can significantly improve survival and recovery outcomes for newborns facing respiratory or circulatory failure.

Preparation, quick action, and effective communication between healthcare providers are key to managing obstetric and neonatal emergencies. Every scenario has its own set of difficulties, and quick action can ensure the mother's and the child's health and safety.

CHAPTER 10: MENTAL HEALTH DISORDERS

Mental health disorders encompass a wide range of conditions that affect an individual's mood, thinking, and behavior. These disorders can significantly impact daily functioning, relationships, physical health, and overall quality of life.

Conditions such as anxiety, depression, and schizophrenia are common, each presenting with unique challenges that require tailored approaches to treatment and management. Mental health is as important as physical health, yet it often faces stigma, which can hinder individuals from seeking help. Understanding mental health disorders, their symptoms, and available interventions is crucial for promoting early detection, effective treatment, and compassionate care. This awareness and knowledge can lead to better outcomes and a more supportive environment for those affected.

Common Disorders:

Mental health disorders can affect individuals in various ways, impacting mood, behavior, thought processes, and overall well-being. Anxiety, depression, and schizophrenia are among the most prevalent mental health conditions, each presenting with distinct characteristics and challenges. Understanding these disorders is essential for effective diagnosis, treatment, and support, as they can significantly influence a person's daily life, relationships, and physical health.

Anxiety Disorders

Anxiety disorders are characterized by excessive worry, fear, or nervousness that interferes with daily activities. While experiencing occasional anxiety is a normal part of life, anxiety disorders involve persistent, overwhelming feelings that go beyond typical stress responses. These disorders include generalized anxiety disorder (GAD), panic disorder, social anxiety disorder, and specific phobias.

Generalized anxiety disorder (GAD) is marked by chronic, excessive worry about various aspects of life, such as work, health, relationships, or daily activities. Individuals with GAD often find it difficult to control their worry and may experience physical symptoms like muscle tension, fatigue, restlessness, irritability, and sleep disturbances. This constant state of anxiety can make it challenging to concentrate, make decisions, or enjoy life.

Panic disorder involves recurrent, unexpected panic attacks—intense periods of fear or discomfort that peak within minutes. Symptoms of a panic attack include heart palpitations, shortness of breath, dizziness, trembling, and a feeling of impending doom. Panic attacks can occur unexpectedly, leading to fear of future attacks and avoidance of situations that may trigger them. This avoidance can limit daily activities and significantly affect an individual's quality of life.

Social anxiety disorder is characterized by an intense fear of social situations where one might feel embarrassed, judged, or scrutinized. This fear can result in avoiding social interactions, public speaking, or situations where the person feels exposed. Individuals with social anxiety may experience physical symptoms like sweating, blushing, trembling, or nausea in social settings, which further reinforces their fear and avoidance behavior.

Management of anxiety disorders typically involves a combination of psychotherapy, medication, and lifestyle changes. Cognitive-behavioral therapy (CBT) is one of the most effective forms of therapy for anxiety, helping individuals identify and change negative thought patterns and behaviors. Medications such as selective serotonin reuptake inhibitors (SSRIs) and benzodiazepines may be prescribed to manage symptoms. Regular physical activity, mindfulness practices, and stress management techniques can also support overall mental health and reduce anxiety.

Depression

Depression, or major depressive disorder (MDD), is a common but serious mental health condition characterized by persistent feelings of sadness, hopelessness, and a loss of interest or pleasure in daily activities. It affects how a person thinks, feels, and behaves, often leading to a variety of emotional and physical problems.

Key symptoms of depression include prolonged periods of sadness, irritability, fatigue, changes in appetite (either increased or decreased), sleep disturbances (insomnia or oversleeping), difficulty concentrating, and feelings of worthlessness or guilt. In severe cases, individuals may have thoughts of self-harm or suicide. The symptoms of depression vary in severity and duration, but they typically persist for at least two weeks, affecting daily functioning and overall quality of life.

Depression can be triggered by various factors, including genetics, brain chemistry imbalances, hormonal changes, chronic medical conditions, trauma, or stressful life events. It often coexists with other mental health disorders, such as anxiety, and can contribute to or result from substance use disorders.

Management of depression involves a multi-faceted approach. Psychotherapy, particularly cognitive-behavioral therapy (CBT) and interpersonal therapy (IPT), is effective in helping individuals understand and manage their thoughts and emotions. Medications such as selective serotonin reuptake inhibitors (SSRIs), serotonin-norepinephrine reuptake inhibitors (SNRIs), or tricyclic antidepressants (TCAs) are commonly prescribed to regulate brain chemistry and alleviate depressive symptoms. Lifestyle changes, including regular exercise, a balanced diet, adequate sleep, and social support, play a crucial role in managing depression. For severe cases, especially where there is a risk of self-harm, interventions such as hospitalization or electroconvulsive therapy (ECT) may be necessary.

Schizophrenia

Schizophrenia is a complex, chronic mental health disorder that affects a person's thinking, behavior, and perception of reality. It typically emerges in late adolescence or early adulthood and has a profound impact on daily functioning. Unlike anxiety or depression, schizophrenia involves psychotic symptoms, which can be severely disabling without proper treatment and support.

Symptoms of schizophrenia fall into three main categories: positive, negative, and cognitive. Positive symptoms include hallucinations (hearing or seeing things that aren't there), delusions (strongly held false beliefs, often of persecution or grandeur), and disorganized thinking (difficulty in organizing thoughts, leading to incoherent speech). Negative symptoms refer to a reduction in normal emotional and behavioral functioning, such as a lack of motivation, social withdrawal, and a diminished ability to experience pleasure (anhedonia). Cognitive symptoms affect memory, attention, and executive functioning, making it hard for individuals to plan, organize, and make decisions.

The exact cause of schizophrenia remains unclear, but it is believed to result from a combination of genetic predisposition, brain chemistry imbalances, and environmental factors such as prenatal exposure to infections or trauma. These factors can alter brain development, affecting the neurotransmitter systems involved in mood, thinking, and perception.

Management of schizophrenia is often lifelong and requires a comprehensive approach. Antipsychotic medications are the cornerstone of treatment, helping to reduce or eliminate psychotic symptoms by regulating neurotransmitters in the brain. Second-generation (atypical) antipsychotics, such as risperidone and olanzapine, are commonly used due to their effectiveness and lower risk of severe side effects compared to first-generation antipsychotics.

In addition to medication, psychosocial interventions are vital. Cognitive-behavioral therapy (CBT) helps individuals develop coping strategies for managing symptoms and challenging delusional thinking. Social skills training and supportive therapy can improve daily functioning, interpersonal relationships, and quality of life. For those experiencing severe or recurrent symptoms, community support services, including case management, vocational rehabilitation, and supervised housing, are essential to facilitate stability and independence.

Anxiety, depression, and schizophrenia each present unique challenges and complexities that can significantly affect an individual's life. Proper diagnosis, early intervention, and a tailored treatment plan involving therapy, medication, lifestyle changes, and social support are essential in managing these disorders. Understanding the nature and impact of these mental health conditions fosters greater compassion and opens up pathways for effective care, ultimately improving outcomes for those affected.

Screening and Diagnostic Tools:

Screening and diagnostic tools are essential in identifying mental health disorders, enabling early intervention and appropriate treatment planning. In clinical settings, tools like the Patient Health Questionnaire-9 (PHQ-9), Generalized Anxiety Disorder-7 (GAD-7), and the Mini- Mental State Examination (MMSE) are commonly used to assess symptoms, determine the severity of mental health conditions, and monitor progress over time. These tools provide valuable insights for healthcare providers to make informed decisions regarding diagnosis and management.

Patient Health Questionnaire-9 (PHQ-9)

The PHQ-9 is a widely used screening tool for assessing the severity of depression. It consists of nine questions that correspond to the diagnostic criteria for major depressive disorder in the Diagnostic and Statistical Manual of Mental Disorders (DSM). Each question asks the individual to rate the frequency of specific depressive symptoms, such as lack of interest in activities, changes in sleep patterns, fatigue, difficulty concentrating, feelings of hopelessness, and thoughts of self-harm, over the past two weeks. Responses are scored on a scale from 0 ("Not at all") to 3 ("Nearly every day"), with a maximum total score of 27.

Scores are interpreted to gauge the severity of depression:

- 0–4: Minimal or none
- 5–9: Mild depression

- 10–14: Moderate depression
- 15–19: Moderately severe depression
- 20–27: Severe depression

A score of 10 or above generally indicates the need for further evaluation and potential intervention. The PHQ-9 is not only helpful in initial screening but also serves as a useful tool for tracking changes in symptom severity over time, providing healthcare providers with a clear picture of a patient's response to treatment.

Generalized Anxiety Disorder-7 (GAD-7)

The GAD-7 is a brief screening tool used to assess the severity of generalized anxiety disorder (GAD). It consists of seven questions that address core symptoms of anxiety, such as excessive worry, restlessness, irritability, muscle tension, and sleep disturbances. Similar to the PHQ-9, individuals rate the frequency of each symptom over the past two weeks on a scale of 0 ("Not at all") to 3 ("Nearly every day"), with a total possible score of 21.

The scoring interpretation helps determine the severity of anxiety:

- 0–4: Minimal anxiety
- 5–9: Mild anxiety
- 10–14: Moderate anxiety
- 15–21: Severe anxiety

A score of 10 or higher indicates clinically significant anxiety, warranting further assessment and possible intervention. The GAD-7 is an effective tool for identifying not only GAD but also other anxiety-related conditions, such as panic disorder and social anxiety disorder. It also assists in monitoring symptom changes, making it valuable for guiding treatment adjustments and evaluating the effectiveness of interventions.

Mini-Mental State Examination (MMSE)

The MMSE is a commonly used tool for assessing cognitive function and screening for cognitive impairment, including conditions like dementia and Alzheimer's disease. The test evaluates various cognitive domains, including orientation, memory, attention, calculation, language, and visuospatial skills. The MMSE consists of 30 points, with different tasks designed to assess specific cognitive abilities.

Examples of tasks include:

- Orientation: Asking the individual to state the current date, time, location, and season.
- Registration: Naming three objects and asking the individual to repeat them.
- Attention and Calculation: Counting backward from 100 by sevens or spelling a word backward.
- Recall: Asking the individual to recall the three objects mentioned earlier.

- Language: Following simple instructions, naming objects, repeating phrases, and writing a sentence.

The MMSE scoring is generally interpreted as follows:

- 24–30: Normal cognitive function
- 18–23: Mild cognitive impairment
- 0–17: Severe cognitive impairment

While the MMSE is not diagnostic on its own, it provides a quick overview of cognitive abilities and can signal the need for further, more comprehensive evaluation. It is especially useful in primary care settings for initial screening and in tracking cognitive changes over time, which can aid in the diagnosis and management of conditions like dementia.

Integrating Screening Tools in Clinical Practice

Using tools like the PHQ-9, GAD-7, and MMSE allows healthcare providers to systematically identify mental health issues, assess their severity, and monitor changes over time. These tools support a structured approach to evaluating mental health, facilitating early diagnosis and the development of tailored treatment plans. By incorporating these screening instruments into regular assessments, clinicians can enhance the quality of mental health care and promote better outcomes for individuals experiencing anxiety, depression, cognitive impairment, or other mental health concerns.

Management Strategies:

Management of mental health disorders requires a comprehensive approach that considers the unique needs of each individual. Key strategies include psychotherapy, pharmacotherapy, and crisis intervention. These methods can be used individually or in combination to provide effective treatment, alleviate symptoms, and improve overall well-being. Addressing mental health conditions in a holistic manner enables patients to achieve better long-term outcomes and enhances their quality of life.

Psychotherapy

Psychotherapy, often referred to as talk therapy, is a cornerstone in the management of mental health disorders such as anxiety, depression, and schizophrenia. It involves working with a trained mental health professional to explore thoughts, feelings, and behaviors, and to develop coping mechanisms and strategies for managing symptoms. There are several types of psychotherapy, each tailored to address specific conditions and individual needs.

Cognitive Behavioral Therapy (CBT) is one of the most widely used forms of psychotherapy, especially for anxiety and depression. It focuses on identifying and challenging negative thought patterns and behaviors that contribute to emotional distress. By reframing these thoughts and adopting healthier behaviors, individuals can break the cycle of anxiety and depression. CBT is structured, goal-oriented, and often short-term, typically lasting between 8 to 20 sessions. Patients learn practical skills for managing stress, improving mood, and coping with difficult situations, making it an effective tool for long-term self-management.

Interpersonal Therapy (IPT) is particularly useful for managing depression. It centers on improving interpersonal relationships and communication patterns, which can significantly affect one's emotional state. By addressing issues such as grief, role transitions, interpersonal conflicts, and social isolation, IPT helps individuals develop healthier relationships and social support networks, which are crucial for recovery.

Dialectical Behavior Therapy (DBT) is another form of therapy, particularly effective for individuals with borderline personality disorder, emotional dysregulation, or self-harm tendencies. DBT combines cognitive-behavioral techniques with mindfulness practices to help individuals manage intense emotions, reduce self-destructive behaviors, and improve interpersonal relationships.

Family Therapy can also be beneficial, especially for individuals with conditions like schizophrenia. Involving family members in therapy helps create a supportive environment, educates them about the disorder, and equips them with strategies to aid in their loved one's recovery.

Pharmacotherapy

Pharmacotherapy, or medication management, is often an essential component in treating mental health disorders. While psychotherapy addresses behavioral and emotional aspects, medications target the underlying neurochemical imbalances associated with conditions such as anxiety, depression, and schizophrenia. The choice of medication depends on the specific disorder, symptom severity, and the patient's overall health.

For anxiety disorders, selective serotonin reuptake inhibitors (SSRIs) like sertraline, fluoxetine, and escitalopram are commonly prescribed. SSRIs work by increasing the levels of serotonin in the brain, a neurotransmitter that plays a key role in regulating mood and anxiety. Other medications such as benzodiazepines (e.g., alprazolam, lorazepam) may be used for short-term relief of acute anxiety symptoms but are typically avoided for long-term use due to the risk of dependency.

In depression, SSRIs and serotonin-norepinephrine reuptake inhibitors (SNRIs) like venlafaxine and duloxetine are the first-line medications. These drugs help alleviate depressive symptoms by balancing neurotransmitter levels. In cases of treatment-resistant depression, other classes of medications, including tricyclic antidepressants (TCAs) and atypical antipsychotics, may be considered.

For schizophrenia, antipsychotic medications are the primary treatment. These include first- generation (typical) antipsychotics like haloperidol and second-generation (atypical) antipsychotics such as risperidone, olanzapine, and aripiprazole. Atypical antipsychotics are often preferred due to their lower risk of severe side effects compared to typical antipsychotics. These medications help manage symptoms such as hallucinations, delusions, and disorganized thinking, enabling patients to function more effectively in daily life. Medication adherence is crucial, as discontinuation can lead to relapse and worsening of symptoms.

Crisis Intervention

Crisis intervention is a critical strategy for managing acute mental health crises, such as severe anxiety or panic attacks, suicidal ideation, and psychotic episodes. These situations require immediate attention to ensure the safety of the individual and those around them. Crisis intervention aims to provide rapid support, stabilize the situation, and guide the individual toward longer-term treatment and care.

In cases of severe anxiety or panic attacks, immediate intervention focuses on creating a calm environment and using grounding techniques to help the individual regain control. Breathing exercises and mindfulness practices can reduce acute symptoms and provide a sense of safety. Providing reassurance and a listening ear can help individuals feel supported during a distressing episode.

When dealing with suicidal ideation or self-harm tendencies, the first step is to assess the risk level by asking direct questions about suicidal thoughts, plans, and access to means. High-risk individuals may need emergency psychiatric care, including hospitalization, to ensure their safety. Crisis hotlines, mental health crisis teams, and emergency services play a vital role in providing immediate support and connecting individuals to professional help.

For psychotic episodes, immediate intervention may involve using de-escalation techniques to reduce agitation and avoid confrontation. In situations where the individual poses a risk to themselves or others, emergency medical services or crisis teams may need to facilitate transport to a hospital or psychiatric facility. In a controlled setting, antipsychotic medications are administered to stabilize symptoms. Once stabilized, the patient can transition to long-term treatment, which includes regular medication management and psychotherapy.

In all forms of crisis intervention, follow-up care is essential. After the acute phase, individuals should be connected with mental health professionals for ongoing support, therapy, and medication management. Crisis plans can be developed to prepare for potential future crises, involving coping strategies, emergency contacts, and a list of support resources.

Combining psychotherapy, pharmacotherapy, and crisis intervention creates a comprehensive approach to managing mental health disorders. This integrated strategy addresses both the emotional and physiological aspects of these conditions, promoting recovery, stability, and an improved quality of life for individuals affected by mental health challenges.

Mental health disorders encompass a wide range of conditions that affect an individual's mood, thinking, and behavior. These disorders can significantly impact daily functioning, relationships, physical health, and overall quality of life. Conditions such as anxiety, depression, and schizophrenia are common, each presenting with unique challenges that require tailored approaches to treatment and management. Mental health is as important as physical health, yet it often faces stigma, which can hinder individuals from seeking help. Understanding mental health disorders, their symptoms, and available interventions is crucial for promoting early detection, effective treatment, and compassionate care. This awareness and knowledge can lead to better outcomes and a more supportive environment for those affected.

CHAPTER 11: ESSENTIAL DIAGNOSTIC TOOLS

Essential diagnostic tools are crucial in assessing and managing a wide range of medical conditions. These tools, including electrocardiogram (ECG) interpretation, basic radiology, and lab tests, provide critical insights into a patient's health. The effective use
of these tools aids in diagnosing diseases, monitoring treatment, and making informed clinical decisions. Accurate interpretation of ECGs, radiological images, and laboratory test results is fundamental for healthcare professionals to deliver quality care.

An electrocardiogram (ECG) is one of the most frequently used diagnostic tools in clinical practice, particularly for assessing heart health. It records the electrical activity of the heart over a set period and offers vital information about heart rate, rhythm, and the overall functioning of the heart. Interpreting an ECG involves understanding the different waveforms that represent specific phases of the cardiac cycle. The P wave reflects atrial contraction, and abnormalities in this wave can signal atrial enlargement or arrhythmias. The QRS complex represents ventricular depolarization, and any changes in its width or height might indicate blockages or issues with the heart's ventricles. The T wave shows ventricular repolarization, and any unusual shapes or inversions may suggest ischemia or electrolyte imbalances. The ST segment is particularly crucial in diagnosing heart attacks; elevations or depressions in this segment indicate myocardial ischemia or infarction. For example, in cases of a heart attack, an ECG can show significant changes such as ST-segment elevation or new Q waves, helping clinicians quickly identify the severity of the cardiac event. Additionally, arrhythmias like atrial fibrillation or tachycardia are easily diagnosed through ECG interpretation by analyzing the heart's rhythm patterns and beat regularity.

Basic radiology also plays an essential role in diagnosing medical conditions across different systems of the body. Radiological imaging includes tools such as X-rays, ultrasound, and computed tomography (CT) scans, which offer visual representations of internal structures. Chest X-rays are commonly used to assess the lungs, heart, and chest wall. They can reveal conditions such as pneumonia, chronic obstructive pulmonary disease (COPD), or heart failure. An enlarged heart, for instance, can be identified through a chest X-ray, which provides clues to possible underlying heart disease. In cases where pneumonia is suspected, chest X-rays show lung infiltrates that confirm infection. Abdominal X-rays, on the other hand, are valuable in diagnosing bowel obstructions, perforations, or kidney stones. For example, dilated loops of the bowel with air-fluid levels visible on an X-ray suggest an intestinal obstruction, while the presence of free air under the diaphragm indicates a perforated ulcer that requires urgent surgical attention. Ultrasound, a non-invasive and widely used imaging tool, provides real-time images of soft tissues and organs such as the liver, kidneys, gallbladder, and reproductive organs. It is commonly used in pregnancy to monitor fetal development, in cardiology to assess heart function, and in emergency medicine to detect conditions like deep vein thrombosis or abdominal aneurysms. Ultrasound's dynamic capabilities make it a versatile tool for evaluating both acute and chronic conditions. CT scans are particularly useful for their detailed cross- sectional images, which help in diagnosing complex conditions like traumatic injuries, tumors, and vascular issues. A CT scan of the brain, for example, is invaluable in the rapid assessment of stroke, allowing clinicians to differentiate between hemorrhagic and ischemic strokes.

Laboratory tests complement imaging and ECGs by providing biochemical data that reflects the internal functioning of the body. A complete blood count (CBC) is a routine test that provides information about red and white blood cells, hemoglobin, hematocrit, and platelets. Abnormalities in these values can indicate a variety of conditions. For instance, low hemoglobin and hematocrit levels suggest anemia, which could result from conditions such as chronic disease, iron deficiency, or bone marrow disorders. Elevated white blood cell counts may point to infections or inflammation. Platelet counts are essential in evaluating clotting disorders, as both low and high counts can lead to bleeding complications or clot formation, respectively. The basic metabolic panel (BMP) includes measurements of electrolytes like sodium, potassium, and chloride, as well as kidney function markers such as blood urea nitrogen (BUN) and creatinine. Abnormal electrolyte levels, such as high potassium or low sodium, indicate disruptions in the body's fluid balance or kidney function. Elevated BUN and creatinine levels suggest impaired kidney function, which requires further investigation. Liver function tests (LFTs) measure enzymes such as alanine transaminase (ALT) and aspartate transaminase (AST), which are markers of liver damage. Elevated levels of these enzymes indicate liver injury, which could stem from hepatitis, cirrhosis, or toxin exposure. Bilirubin, another component of liver function tests, helps diagnose jaundice and bile duct obstructions.

The coagulation profile, including prothrombin time (PT), activated partial thromboplastin time (aPTT), and the international normalized ratio (INR), assesses the blood's ability to clot. Prolonged clotting times may indicate bleeding disorders, liver disease, or the effects of anticoagulant therapy. Thyroid function tests, which include measurements of thyroid-stimulating hormone (TSH) and free thyroxine (T4), are crucial in diagnosing thyroid disorders. Elevated TSH with low free T4 levels suggests hypothyroidism, while low TSH with high free T4 levels indicates hyperthyroidism.

Incorporating these essential diagnostic tools into clinical practice is fundamental for making accurate diagnoses, monitoring disease progression, and guiding effective treatment plans. The integration of ECG interpretation, radiological imaging, and lab test results allows healthcare professionals to build a comprehensive picture of a patient's health status, leading to better outcomes and improved patient care. By mastering these tools, clinicians can make informed decisions that enhance patient safety and the quality of healthcare delivery.

Physical Examination Techniques

Physical examination techniques are vital components of patient assessment, providing direct, immediate insights into a patient's health. Effective physical examination helps identify abnormalities, monitor disease progression, and guide further diagnostic testing. Key areas of focus include the cardiovascular, respiratory, and neurological systems, as each presents specific signs and symptoms that can be detected through careful examination. Mastery of these techniques allows healthcare providers to make more accurate diagnoses and develop targeted management plans.

In examining the cardiovascular system, the clinician assesses the heart and blood vessels for signs of circulatory health or potential cardiac conditions. The process begins with general inspection, where the patient is observed for signs such as cyanosis (bluish skin discoloration indicating poor oxygenation), pallor, and edema, particularly in the lower extremities, which may suggest heart failure. Checking the jugular venous pressure (JVP) is crucial for assessing the heart's right side function. Elevated JVP can indicate right heart failure or fluid overload, common in conditions like congestive heart failure. Palpation follows, where the healthcare provider feels for the apical impulse, typically located at the fifth intercostal space on the left midclavicular line. A displaced apical impulse may indicate an enlarged heart or ventricular hypertrophy.

Auscultation, using a stethoscope, is a critical step in the cardiovascular exam. The provider listens for heart sounds, focusing on the four key areas: aortic, pulmonic, tricuspid, and mitral regions. The primary heart sounds, S1 (the "lub") and S2 (the "dub"), represent the closing of the heart valves during the cardiac cycle. Abnormal heart sounds, such as murmurs, rubs, or gallops, can signal underlying conditions. For example, murmurs indicate turbulent blood flow, which might result from valve abnormalities like stenosis or regurgitation. Additional heart sounds, such as an S3 or S4, can suggest heart failure or other cardiac abnormalities. Peripheral pulses, including the radial, carotid, femoral, and dorsalis pedis, are also palpated to assess their strength and regularity, providing further clues about cardiac output and vascular health.

The respiratory system examination focuses on evaluating the lungs and chest wall. It begins with inspection, where the healthcare provider observes the patient's breathing pattern, rate, and effort. Signs such as the use of accessory muscles, nasal flaring, or pursed-lip breathing may indicate respiratory distress or chronic obstructive pulmonary disease (COPD). The shape and symmetry of the chest are assessed, looking for abnormalities like barrel chest (commonly seen in COPD) or pectus excavatum (sunken chest). Palpation involves feeling the chest wall for tenderness, crepitus (a crackling sensation indicating air in the subcutaneous tissue), or asymmetrical chest expansion, which may suggest a pneumothorax or pleural effusion.

Percussion of the chest provides information about the underlying lung tissue. The examiner taps on the chest wall and listens to the sound produced. A resonant sound is normal, while dullness can indicate fluid, as seen in pneumonia or pleural effusion, and hyperresonance may suggest air trapping, such as in emphysema or a pneumothorax. Auscultation is performed using a stethoscope to listen to breath sounds across various areas of the lungs. Normal breath sounds include vesicular breathing over most lung fields, while abnormal sounds, like wheezes, crackles, or stridor, may indicate obstructive airway disease, fluid in the lungs, or upper airway obstruction, respectively. Wheezing suggests narrowed airways, often found in asthma or bronchitis, while crackles (rales) may indicate fluid accumulation, as seen in heart failure or pneumonia.

A thorough neurological examination assesses the patient's nervous system, focusing on mental status, cranial nerves, motor function, sensation, coordination, and reflexes. The examination begins with an assessment of the patient's level of consciousness, orientation (to time, place, and person), and cognitive abilities, such as memory and speech. Any abnormalities in mental status may point to conditions affecting the brain, such as stroke, encephalopathy, or neurodegenerative diseases.

The cranial nerve examination involves evaluating all twelve cranial nerves. For instance, testing the optic nerve (cranial nerve II) assesses visual acuity and field, while the oculomotor, trochlear, and abducens nerves (cranial nerves III, IV, and VI) control eye movements. Impairment in these nerves can suggest neurological conditions like multiple sclerosis or increased intracranial pressure. Examination of the facial nerve (cranial nerve VII) includes checking for facial symmetry, which may reveal signs of a stroke or Bell's palsy. Testing the gag reflex and uvula movement assesses the glossopharyngeal and vagus nerves (cranial nerves IX and X), providing clues to brainstem function.

Motor function is evaluated by testing muscle strength, tone, and coordination. The healthcare provider asks the patient to perform specific movements, such as pushing against resistance or walking in a straight line, to assess strength and balance. Abnormalities like muscle weakness, atrophy, or tremors can indicate neurological conditions affecting the motor cortex, spinal cord, or peripheral nerves. Reflexes are tested using a reflex hammer to strike tendons in areas like the knee (patellar reflex) and ankle (Achilles reflex). Abnormal reflex responses, such as hyperreflexia or hyporeflexia, can help localize lesions within the nervous system. For example, hyperreflexia often suggests upper motor neuron involvement, while hyporeflexia indicates lower motor neuron or peripheral nerve damage.

The sensory examination involves assessing the patient's ability to perceive light touch, pain, temperature, vibration, and proprioception (sense of body position). Deficits in sensation can indicate damage to sensory pathways, including peripheral nerves, the spinal cord, or the brain. Additionally, coordination is assessed through tasks such as finger-to-nose or heel-to-shin movements, which help identify cerebellar dysfunction or other neurological impairments.

Through careful physical examination techniques across the cardiovascular, respiratory, and neurological systems, healthcare providers gather essential information about a patient's condition. This hands-on assessment, when combined with clinical history and diagnostic tools, leads to a more accurate diagnosis and better management strategies for the patient's health.

Tips for Efficient and Effective Clinical Assessment

Conducting a clinical assessment efficiently and effectively is crucial in providing high-quality patient care. A thorough yet streamlined assessment helps identify the patient's key health issues, guides diagnostic decisions, and informs treatment strategies. Given the often-limited time healthcare providers have with patients, optimizing the assessment process is essential. Here are some practical tips for conducting an efficient and effective clinical assessment.

Preparation is the first step toward an effective assessment. Before entering the examination room, take a few moments to review the patient's medical history, recent test results, and any notes from previous visits. This background information helps focus the assessment on relevant areas, allowing for a more targeted and productive examination. It also ensures that you have a context for any new symptoms or findings, which can speed up the diagnostic process.

Starting the assessment with a focused yet open-ended questioning approach is key. Begin with broad questions like, "What brings you in today?" to allow the patient to share their concerns. As the patient describes their symptoms, listen attentively and identify key details that require further exploration. Once the main issues are outlined, use more specific, closed-ended questions to clarify and gather detailed information about the symptoms' onset, duration, severity, and any associated factors. This approach ensures that you obtain the necessary information without deviating into less relevant areas.

While taking the patient's history, maintain a structured flow. For example, start with the chief complaint, then move to the history of present illness, followed by past medical history, medication use, family history, and social history. Keeping a consistent order minimizes the risk of missing important information and helps the patient understand what to expect next. This structure also facilitates a smooth transition to the physical examination, as you can easily connect reported symptoms with specific examination techniques.

During the physical examination, prioritize the most relevant systems based on the patient's history and presenting symptoms. For example, if a patient presents with chest pain, a cardiovascular and respiratory examination should take precedence. Conduct a general inspection first, looking for any obvious signs such as distress, abnormal posture, or skin changes. This brief overview provides initial clues that guide the focus of the detailed examination.

When examining specific systems, use a systematic approach to maximize efficiency. For the cardiovascular system, for instance, begin with inspection, then proceed to palpation, auscultation, and finally assess peripheral pulses. This structured sequence ensures that no step is skipped, reduces redundancy, and allows for a comprehensive evaluation within a limited timeframe.

Using the proper techniques during the physical examination is crucial for accuracy. Ensure that you have the necessary tools, such as a stethoscope, reflex hammer, and otoscope, readily available and in good working condition. Proper use of these tools not only enhances the accuracy of findings but also demonstrates professionalism and thoroughness to the patient, fostering trust and cooperation. For example, when using a stethoscope for cardiac auscultation, listen to all four key areas—mitral, tricuspid, aortic, and pulmonic—while varying pressure to capture both high and low-frequency heart sounds. This careful technique can detect subtle murmurs or abnormal heart sounds that might otherwise be missed.

Time management is an integral part of an efficient assessment. Allocate time appropriately based on the complexity of the patient's condition. For patients with multiple or chronic conditions, it may be helpful to address the most pressing issue first, ensuring it receives adequate attention. In follow-up visits, quickly review the status of known conditions before addressing any new symptoms. This prioritization allows for a more focused examination, reserving detailed evaluations for areas that most directly impact the patient's current health status.

Communication is key throughout the assessment process. Explain each step of the examination to the patient in simple, clear language to keep them informed and engaged. For example, say, "I'm going to listen to your lungs now to check for any abnormal sounds." This transparency reduces anxiety, encourages cooperation, and may provide additional information as the patient may reveal more about their symptoms when they understand what you are checking. Additionally, regularly check in with the patient during the assessment by asking questions like, "Does this cause any discomfort?" to gather real-time feedback and ensure the patient's comfort.

Document findings efficiently and accurately as soon as possible, preferably during or immediately after the examination. Use concise notes that focus on key positive and negative findings relevant to the patient's condition. For instance, document significant observations like "clear lung sounds bilaterally" or "no abdominal tenderness." Clear and structured documentation supports continuity of care, assists in future assessments, and facilitates communication with other healthcare professionals.

An effective assessment includes knowing when to seek additional diagnostic tests or specialist consultations. If initial findings point toward specific conditions that require more detailed evaluation, such as imaging studies for suspected fractures or lab tests for metabolic imbalances, order these tests promptly to avoid delays in diagnosis and treatment. When the assessment reveals complex or unclear findings, referring the patient to a specialist can provide further insights and ensure comprehensive care.

By implementing these tips, healthcare providers can perform clinical assessments that are both thorough and time-efficient. This approach ensures that patients receive the best possible care, with accurate diagnoses and timely, tailored interventions based on a clear understanding of their health status.

CHAPTER 12: SIMPLIFIED CASE STUDIES

This section on simplified case studies aims to bridge theory and practice, illustrating how clinical assessment, diagnostic tools, and management strategies are applied in real-world scenarios. These cases provide practical insights into handling common and complex health conditions, helping to refine diagnostic skills and clinical decision-making. By examining different patient presentations, you will gain a deeper understanding of how to identify symptoms, interpret diagnostic findings, and develop effective treatment plans. These cases are designed to simplify intricate medical concepts, making them accessible and relevant for healthcare professionals at various levels of experience. Through these practical examples, you'll learn how to approach clinical challenges systematically and efficiently.

Case Scenarios for Practice:

Exploring case scenarios provides invaluable practice for healthcare professionals, offering insights into the clinical approach needed to address acute and life-threatening conditions. These scenarios illustrate how to recognize symptoms, interpret diagnostic findings, and implement appropriate interventions. The following cases focus on cardiac arrest, acute asthma, and diabetic ketoacidosis (DKA), highlighting the steps required to manage these emergencies effectively.

In a cardiac arrest scenario, a patient suddenly collapses in the emergency department. The patient is unresponsive, with no detectable pulse or breathing. Immediate action is crucial. Begin by activating the emergency response system and initiating cardiopulmonary resuscitation (CPR). Early CPR and defibrillation are key to increasing the chances of survival. Assess the heart rhythm using an automated external defibrillator (AED) or a cardiac monitor. If ventricular fibrillation (VF) or pulseless ventricular tachycardia (VT) is identified, administer a shock as soon as possible and continue CPR. Advanced Cardiac Life Support (ACLS) protocols should be followed, which include the administration of epinephrine every 3-5 minutes and considering other reversible causes, such as hypoxia, hypovolemia, or electrolyte imbalances (the "H's and T's"). Throughout this process, monitoring the patient's response is vital. For example, if the rhythm converts to a normal sinus rhythm with a palpable pulse, shift focus to post-resuscitation care, which includes securing the airway, optimizing blood pressure, and identifying the underlying cause of the arrest to prevent recurrence. This case demonstrates the importance of rapid intervention, adherence to guidelines, and multidisciplinary teamwork in managing cardiac arrest.

In an acute asthma scenario, a young adult presents to the clinic with severe shortness of breath, wheezing, and chest tightness. The patient's respiratory rate is elevated, and they are using accessory muscles to breathe, indicating respiratory distress. Auscultation reveals diffuse wheezing throughout the lung fields. Immediate management focuses on opening the airways and improving oxygenation. Administer high-flow oxygen to maintain adequate oxygen saturation levels, followed by short-acting bronchodilators like albuterol delivered via a nebulizer or metered-dose inhaler with a spacer. Corticosteroids, such as oral prednisone or intravenous methylprednisolone, are given to reduce airway inflammation. Assess peak expiratory flow (PEF) to gauge the severity of the obstruction. In severe cases, where the patient is unable to speak in full sentences or has a PEF less than 50% of the predicted value, escalation of care is required. This may include intravenous magnesium sulfate as a bronchodilator and continuous monitoring for signs of impending respiratory failure, such as altered mental status or decreasing oxygen levels. If the patient does not respond to initial treatment, consider transferring them to a higher level of care, such as the intensive care unit (ICU), for possible intubation and mechanical ventilation. This case illustrates the need for prompt assessment, aggressive treatment, and careful monitoring in managing acute asthma exacerbations.

In a diabetic ketoacidosis (DKA) scenario, a middle-aged patient with type 1 diabetes presents to the emergency department with symptoms of nausea, vomiting, abdominal pain, and rapid, deep breathing (Kussmaul respiration). The patient reports polyuria, polydipsia, and recent non-compliance with insulin therapy.

Initial assessment reveals dehydration, tachycardia, and a fruity odor on the breath, suggestive of ketone production. Obtain blood glucose, electrolyte, and blood gas measurements to confirm the diagnosis. A blood glucose level of over 250 mg/dL, low bicarbonate levels, elevated anion gap, and the presence of ketones in the blood or urine indicate DKA. Management begins with fluid resuscitation using intravenous normal saline to correct dehydration and restore circulatory volume. Insulin therapy is initiated to reduce blood glucose levels and suppress ketone production. Administer intravenous regular insulin with frequent monitoring of blood glucose and potassium levels, as insulin therapy can drive potassium into cells, leading to hypokalemia. Supplement potassium as needed to maintain normal serum levels. As the blood glucose approaches 200 mg/dL, switch to a solution containing dextrose to prevent hypoglycemia and continue insulin therapy until ketonemia resolves and the patient can tolerate oral intake. Throughout treatment, monitor electrolytes, blood gases, and urine output to guide adjustments in therapy. This case highlights the importance of a systematic approach in managing DKA, focusing on fluid and electrolyte balance, insulin administration, and close monitoring to prevent complications.

These scenarios emphasize the critical importance of recognizing signs and symptoms, acting promptly with appropriate interventions, and continuously monitoring patients to adapt treatment as needed. They also demonstrate the significance of following established clinical protocols in managing emergencies such as cardiac arrest, acute asthma, and DKA. By practicing these case scenarios, healthcare professionals can develop a structured approach to acute care, enhancing their ability to manage complex situations effectively.

Clinical Decision Points:

Clinical decision-making is at the heart of effective patient care, especially when managing acute conditions like cardiac arrest, acute asthma, and diabetic ketoacidosis (DKA). In these critical scenarios, rapid diagnosis, immediate interventions, and structured follow-up care are essential to ensure the best possible outcomes for patients. Each step involves assessing the situation, acting quickly with appropriate treatments, and planning for long-term management to prevent recurrence or complications.

Rapid diagnosis forms the foundation of successful intervention. In cases like cardiac arrest, recognizing the signs—such as loss of consciousness, absence of pulse, and cessation of breathing—is crucial. Quick confirmation using tools like an automated external defibrillator (AED) or cardiac monitor helps identify the type of arrest, whether it's ventricular fibrillation (VF), ventricular tachycardia (VT), or asystole. Similarly, in acute asthma, the presence of severe shortness of breath, wheezing, and use of accessory muscles signals the need for immediate assessment. Using tools like a peak flow meter to gauge airflow limitation aids in determining the severity of the exacerbation. For DKA, initial assessment includes checking blood glucose levels, serum ketones, electrolytes, and blood gases. Signs like rapid, deep breathing (Kussmaul respirations), dehydration, and fruity-scented breath indicate the urgency of the condition. These rapid diagnostic steps enable healthcare professionals to initiate prompt and targeted interventions.

Immediate interventions are the next critical phase in managing these acute scenarios. For cardiac arrest, initiating cardiopulmonary resuscitation (CPR) within seconds of recognition is vital. Alongside CPR, the use of defibrillation for shockable rhythms like VF or VT can significantly improve survival rates. Administration of drugs like epinephrine is integrated into Advanced Cardiac Life Support (ACLS) protocols to support the heart's function during resuscitation. In the case of acute asthma, administering high-flow oxygen and bronchodilators, such as albuterol, helps to relieve airway obstruction. Corticosteroids are then added to reduce inflammation in the airways. In severe cases where the patient is not responding to initial treatments, intravenous magnesium sulfate may be used to further open the airways. If the patient's condition deteriorates, intubation and mechanical ventilation may be necessary. For DKA, the immediate goal is to correct fluid deficits and high blood glucose levels. Intravenous fluid resuscitation with normal saline is the first step to address dehydration and stabilize circulation. Alongside fluid therapy, insulin administration is crucial to decrease blood glucose and halt ketone production. Frequent monitoring of electrolytes, particularly potassium, guides the adjustment of therapy, as insulin can lower potassium levels, potentially leading to life-threatening hypokalemia. These immediate interventions are lifesaving, and they need to be tailored to the patient's response to treatment.

Follow-up care is an equally vital component of patient management, as it focuses on preventing recurrence, managing long-term health, and ensuring recovery. In cardiac arrest survivors, follow-up care involves identifying and treating the underlying cause, which might include coronary artery disease, arrhythmias, or electrolyte imbalances. This may require further cardiac evaluation, such as an echocardiogram or cardiac catheterization, to assess heart function and structure. Medications, lifestyle modifications, and in some cases, procedures like the implantation of a defibrillator may be recommended to prevent future cardiac events. Additionally, patients often need psychological support to cope with the emotional impact of experiencing a life-threatening event.

For asthma patients, follow-up care focuses on preventing future exacerbations. After stabilizing an acute asthma attack, clinicians review and optimize the patient's asthma management plan, which includes regular use of inhaled corticosteroids and bronchodilators. Education about avoiding triggers, proper inhaler technique, and recognizing early signs of worsening asthma are key components of long-term care. Scheduled follow-up visits allow for monitoring lung function and adjusting treatment as needed. In some cases, referral to an asthma specialist for further evaluation and management may be beneficial.

In the context of DKA, follow-up care involves both short-term and long-term management strategies. After the acute episode resolves, patients require careful monitoring of blood glucose levels, electrolyte balance, and kidney function. Education on insulin therapy, blood glucose self-monitoring, and dietary adjustments is crucial to prevent recurrence. For patients with type 1 diabetes, regular follow-up with an endocrinologist helps optimize insulin regimens and address lifestyle factors that influence glucose control. Patients are also educated about recognizing early symptoms of hyperglycemia and ketosis, enabling them to seek prompt treatment before DKA develops again.

These clinical decision points—rapid diagnosis, immediate interventions, and structured follow-up care—form the core of effective patient management. By quickly identifying the problem, acting decisively, and planning for long-term recovery and prevention, healthcare professionals can greatly improve outcomes for patients facing acute medical crises. This holistic approach not only addresses the immediate life-threatening issues but also supports the patient in maintaining health and preventing future complications.

BONUSES

SCAN QR FOR DOWNLOAD

APPENDIX

The appendix serves as a valuable resource for healthcare professionals, providing quick access to essential information that supports efficient clinical decision-making. In this section, you will find reference tables for common conditions and drug dosages, along
with key diagnostic criteria and clinical pathways to guide assessment and treatment.

Reference Tables: Common Conditions and Drug Dosages

For swift identification and management of frequent medical conditions, the quick reference tables below summarize key aspects of some common issues encountered in clinical practice.

Hypertension:

- Normal Blood Pressure: <120/80 mm Hg
- Stage 1 Hypertension: 130-139/80-89 mm Hg
- Stage 2 Hypertension: ≥140/90 mm Hg

First-Line Medications:

- ACE Inhibitors: Lisinopril, starting dose: 10 mg once daily
- Calcium Channel Blockers: Amlodipine, starting dose: 5 mg once daily
- Thiazide Diuretics: Hydrochlorothiazide, starting dose: 12.5-25 mg once daily

Diabetes Management:

Diagnostic Criteria:

- Fasting Blood Glucose: ≥126 mg/dL
- HbA1c: ≥6.5%
- Oral Glucose Tolerance Test: 2-hour plasma glucose ≥200 mg/dL

Insulin Dosages:

- Short-acting (Regular): Initial dose: 0.1-0.2 units/kg per meal
- Long-acting (Glargine): Initial dose: 0.2-0.3 units/kg per day

Oral Medications:

- Metformin: Starting dose: 500 mg once or twice daily, maximum dose: 2,000-2,500 mg daily

Asthma:

Severity Classification:

- Mild Intermittent: Symptoms <2 days/week, normal PEF ≥80% of predicted
- Mild Persistent: Symptoms >2 days/week, normal PEF ≥80% of predicted
- Moderate Persistent: Daily symptoms, PEF 60-80% of predicted
- Severe Persistent: Continuous symptoms, PEF <60% of predicted

Treatment Dosages:

- Short-acting Beta Agonists (SABA): Albuterol, 2 puffs every 4-6 hours as needed
- Inhaled Corticosteroids: Budesonide, starting dose: 200-400 mcg twice daily
- These tables serve as a concise overview for quick reference, enabling clinicians to make informed decisions during patient encounters.
- Key Diagnostic Criteria and Clinical Pathways

Accurate diagnosis is central to effective patient care. The following criteria and pathways streamline the assessment and management process:

Acute Myocardial Infarction (AMI):

Diagnostic Criteria:

- Chest Pain: Sudden onset, lasting >20 minutes, radiating to the arm, jaw, or back.
- ECG Changes: ST-segment elevation or depression, T-wave inversion.

- Biomarkers: Elevated troponin levels, indicating myocardial damage.

Clinical Pathway: Administer the MONA protocol (Morphine, Oxygen, Nitroglycerin, Aspirin) immediately, followed by reperfusion therapy (thrombolytics or PCI) based on the patient's presentation and time of symptom onset.

Diabetic Ketoacidosis (DKA):

Diagnostic Criteria:

- Blood Glucose: >250 mg/dL
- Arterial pH: <7.3
- Serum Bicarbonate: <18 mEq/L
- Ketones: Positive in serum or urine

Clinical Pathway: Initiate fluid resuscitation with normal saline, followed by insulin infusion. Monitor electrolytes, especially potassium, and adjust treatment as necessary until the patient is stabilized and blood glucose and ketone levels are within normal ranges.

Stroke (Cerebrovascular Accident):

Diagnostic Criteria:

- Clinical Presentation: Sudden weakness, facial drooping, difficulty speaking, vision changes.
- Imaging: Non-contrast CT scan to distinguish between ischemic and hemorrhagic stroke.
- Clinical Pathway: For ischemic stroke within the therapeutic window, consider thrombolytic therapy with tissue plasminogen activator (tPA). For hemorrhagic stroke, focus on blood pressure control, monitoring for increased intracranial pressure, and surgical intervention if indicated.

This appendix provides a streamlined, at-a-glance guide for healthcare professionals, facilitating prompt and appropriate responses to various clinical scenarios. By having quick access to diagnostic criteria, treatment dosages, and management pathways, clinicians can enhance the quality and efficiency of patient care in a variety of settings.

Made in the USA
Monee, IL
17 November 2024